# Gutsy

## The Food-Mood Method to Revitalize Your Health Beyond Conventional Medicine

# NAN FOSTER

It takes a GUTSY woman to cure herself! And Nan Foster does just that in GUTSY: The Food-Mood Method to Revitalize Your Health Beyond Conventional Medicine. If you're feeling stressed, fatigued, lonely, irritable or sad, join Nan as she walks you through the steps that cured her and helps you diagnose what can cure you, too. From discovering food sensitivities with a 21-day food elimination guide to discovering joy and cooking and shopping with ease, Nan's personal story and tools for writing yours will make you shriek "I'll have what SHE'S having!"

–Sue Brown, author, *Simply Sugar Free:*
*Six Simple Steps to Conquer Sugar Addiction*

Nan Foster uses her considerable expertise in coaching to create an intelligent, holistic, refreshing new roadmap for increasing aliveness and reversing ubiquitous and poorly understood chronic conditions. Her approach is smart, pragmatic and sophisticated, yet user-friendly. Most important, her methods work and her recipes are delightful for the soul-mind-heart-body.

–Anne de Lovinfosse, Ph.D., Licensed
psychologist, coach, yoga nidra teacher

Gutsy is written by Nan Foster, a graduate of the Institute for Integrative Nutrition, where she completed a cutting edge curriculum in nutrition and health coaching taught by the world's leading experts in health and wellness. I recommend you read this book and be in touch with Nan to see how she can help you successfully achieve your goals.

–Joshua Rosenthal, MScEd, Founder/
Director, Institute for Integrative Nutrition

**Gutsy**
The Food-Mood Method to Revitalize Your
Health Beyond Conventional Medicine

Nan Foster
June, 2016

**Gutsy**
The Food-Mood Method to Revitalize Your
Health Beyond Conventional Medicine

Copyright © 2016 by Nan Foster

The content of this book is for general instruction only. Each person's physical, emotional, and spiritual condition is unique. The instruction in this book is not intended to replace or interrupt the reader's relationship with a physician or other professional. Please consult your doctor for matters pertaining to your specific health and diet.

To contact the author, visit www.nanfosterhealth.com

**ISBN-13: 978-1530373901**
**ISBN-10: 1530373905**

Printed in the United States of America

Cover photo credits:
Lightspring/Shutterstock.com; Pinkyone/Shutterstock.com; SOMMAI/ Shutterstock.com; iStock.com/phototake

Primary Food(s) and Secondary Food(s): © 2005 Integrative Nutrition Inc. (used with permission)

Illustration credit: Jamey Ekins/Shutterstock.com

This book is dedicated to my most intimate support system, my incredible family. My husband Rob, my sons, Matt and Dylan, and my father Bob, you are the sustenance that feeds my soul. Thank you for staying curious and open-minded. Mostly, thank you all for loving me the way you do. Lastly, to my mother, Ruth, who was passionate and creative with food, and who still inspires me every day.

# ACKNOWLEDGMENTS

I am so grateful to the generous people who time-traveled back to the beginnings of their health journeys to share their beautiful stories of healing throughout the book: Daniel Goodman, Ardith Plimack, Hannah Plimack, Debbie Toizer as well as Deacon Carpenter, Clinical Ayurvedic Specialist, and owner of YogaONE in Santa Rosa, CA. To my amazing reviewers who committed their time to read, digest, comment, edit and provide their wisdom: Ricka Baker, Elizabeth DeRuff, Rob Foster, MD, Laurie House, Ardith Plimack, and Janice Zunde, I so appreciate you.

Thank you also to my very talented editor Daryn Eller, and to the encouraging book instructors at the Institute for Integrative Nutrition® (IIN®), Lindsey Smith, Sue Brown, Kathleen DiChiara, and Marissa Leigh whose wisdom and guidance made this book possible. And gratitude to IIN® founder, visionary and devoted teacher, Joshua Rosenthal whose program and philosophy helped me find my true calling as a health coach.

# Table of Contents

# Introduction

Just a few short years ago I was what you might call down and out. Not in the fiscal sense, but in the *physical* sense. The emotional and spiritual sense, too. I was lonely, irritable, and sad. Then, on the heels of all that negativity came odd and debilitating symptoms of acne, joint pain, muscle aches, numb tongue and toe, brain fog, and a mild sore throat. Like most people, I initially thought that a pill might cure these problems, but then I hesitated. Wasn't there a more natural and maybe better road to wellness? It turns out there was. I felt hopeful, even bold, determined to find relief beyond a conventional approach. In fact, the simple shifts in diet I made and the new mind-body awareness I developed did more to heal me than any pharmaceutical could. It was an epiphany and it changed my entire life. Now I want to present you with the tools that will change your life too.

Are you interested in learning how to diminish the flames of destructive inflammation, and feel balanced and energized? Perhaps you have been diagnosed with an inflammatory or auto-immune disease such as diabetes, heart disease, arthritis, multiple sclerosis, lupus, Hashimoto's thyroiditis (hypothyroidism), Graves' disease, irritable bowel syndrome (IBS), Sjogren's, fibromyalgia, Raynaud's, rosacea, eczema, psoriasis, or another of the 80-plus autoimmune diseases. Don't despair. A diagnosis is not necessarily the last stop on your health journey. In fact, it can be just the bombshell you need to become aware, get motivated, and adopt some healthy new habits to heal the root cause of the disease. What we have been taught to think of as "disease"–something, its name implies, that is set in stone–can actually be undone.

Maybe you have never been diagnosed with a disease, but *you* know that you feel awful all the time. You're achy. Your stomach often hurts. You're low energy, grumpy, depressed. Well, believe me when I tell you that, through dedication and consistency, it is possible to alleviate all those symptoms of illness. You can achieve your goals–whether those goals are to find relief from aches and pain, have more vitality for your kids or job, to develop a renewed sexual connection with your significant other, or simply to better your overall wellbeing–and you can do it without being beholden to a bag full of pills. Instead, you can affect your health and outlook by simply changing what you eat and how you think.

So if there is a part of you that suspects and hopes there must be more to good health than pharmaceuticals, and if you are curious, even skeptical about the intentions and self-interests of the pharmaceutical industry, then you have come to the right place. This is not to say that traditional medicine doesn't have a role in good health. I'm married to a doctor! For acute and emergency situations like cancer and broken bones, modern medicine can offer us remarkable relief and treatment. However, for chronic conditions with such symptoms as inflammation, pain, and digestive issues, physicians are frequently quick to diagnose without looking deeper for the cause. That leaves it up to us to go beyond diagnosis to pursue the best course of action. In this book I will show you how. On the following pages, you will find simple steps to:

- Reduce inflammation
- Impact gene expression
- Reverse so-called diseases
- Improve nutrient absorption
- Bolster immunity
- Positively affect your brain and mood

## Why I'm So Sure You Can Heal Yourself

Have you ever felt that simply waking up each day was an effort? That the carefree, younger you was long gone? That the universe didn't have your back? That was my perspective when I began feeling unwell. And though I desperately wanted to feel energetic and abundant with optimism and love, instead my cup seemed half-full. I had to depend on the energy of others to lift me up. Little did I know that a disease process was brewing inside of me. Nor did I yet know that it is actually possible to reverse many diseases by addressing the imbalance and inflammation that causes them in the first place. What I came to learn was that the key to health lies in the foods and thoughts we digest every day.

Let me explain. *Straightforward, no-nonsense, goal-oriented, unfiltered New Yorker finds health and self-love in California, embracing New Age, gluten-free, meditative, organic lifestyle.* If you had told me 20 years ago that this would be my destiny—or that I would one day become a certified health coach through the Institute of Integrative Nutrition®—I would have laughed at you. Without a crystal ball, it took a leap of faith to relocate away from my beloved New York City where fashion, finance, and forthright commiseration take center stage. At the time, I was a new mom, following my husband across the country, leaving loved ones behind. It made me feel unsettled, lonely, and stressed. Resistance to settling in the San Francisco Bay Area, with its stunning scenery, year-round fitness, and a ubiquitous "chill" outlook (can you imagine rejecting that?), made my health begin to suffer. I was a sad sack. A negative attitude, anger, and irritability threw me so far out of whack that it manifested in my body. All the symptoms I mentioned earlier—acne, joint pain, muscle aches, numb tongue and toe, brain fog and mild sore throat—were clues I later learned were indicative of inflammation and an autoimmune disease.

On a hunch and a prayer, I set out to research all I could to reverse my symptoms naturally, without medication. I turned to friends. I scoured the Internet for information. I took workshops on mind-body practices. And what I discovered surprised me with its simplicity: I needed a food-mood makeover. Experimenting with West Coast advancements in nutrition and self-help, I began to carve a pathway to health, and to create a new life brimming with forgiveness, gratitude, and joy.

In the past, I had lived a far less healthful life. I thrived under the late nights and demands of college and the high-stress lifestyle of living and working in New York City. I delighted in the blissful ignorance of eating and drinking whatever I pleased. But like a car in need of an oil change, I needed to refresh my body and detox the gunk. By heeding a nasty food intolerance and cleaning up my diet, adding healthful forms of exercise to my routine, then finding gratitude, I proved to myself that lifestyle choices affect our wellbeing and even our genes through the main engines of our health—our minds and our guts. In my case, a simple food elimination process and an outlook makeover illuminated what was causing my weird aches and pains and provided the awareness I needed to reverse an autoimmune disease. Yes, reverse!

The stresses of food sensitivities, toxins, and negative thoughts and beliefs stoke the fire of inflammation; cause imbalances in our gut microbiome (the balance of good and bad bacteria in the digestive system), immunity, and hormones; turn genes on and off; and lead to a cascade of other health issues. Fortunately, digestive system health, nutrition, and the power of the mind are now well studied and understood among scientific communities, allowing us to find solutions to the problems so many of us face.

I have felt especially lucky to have cutting-edge California know-how at my fingertips—especially as more health challenges have come my way. Next up: osteoporosis, and most recently, pre-diabetes. As each health challenge has occurred, after stressing and taking some deep breaths, I've reversed each condition with simple natural changes, reinforcing the fact that healing is possible. I am grateful to both coasts for opening my eyes to their yin and yang sensibilities, one edgy, the other calm, and to family and friends who supported me along the way. Now, after having studied hundreds of dietary theories, looking at the scientific research on the impact of clean eating and positive psychology on balancing body and mind, *and* vastly improving my own wellbeing, I am excited to share these lessons with you. What you'll find in this book are the most current approaches to food and mood—in other words, everything you need to help you regain good health.

There's no reason to accept suffering with symptoms as your new "normal." Once you start the Food-Mood Method I outline in Chapter 6, you'll find pleasure and relief in new places. Deprivation is not invited to this party, but neither is overindulgence. Certainly, the lure of junky comfort foods can be strong. I get it. The mere thought of modifying the diet can rattle us: What will I turn to when I'm stressed or tired? In fact, once we delete the junk from our diets, real food that formerly paled in comparison to sweet, salty processed flavors starts to taste sublime. What's more, real food provides nutrients that curtail cravings so that, once you switch up your diet, you will actually crave junk less and desire wholesome food more. It was a sparkling sunny day at the farmer's market when I tasted my first organic, fresh-picked white peach. The heady floral scent and dripping essence of sweet delight were the perfect antidote to any thoughts of gluten and sugar deprivation. This is nature's way of delighting us, reminding us of the pleasure of eating from the land, the very clue we need to achieve wellness.

## Making the Commitment

I won't sugar coat this: It takes focus, determination, and effort to uncover your root causes and make health-supportive changes. Maybe you are feeling slightly resistant to change—you're too busy; it's too much effort; a pill is quick and easy. But look at it this way: With each small step of change, you are that much closer to your goal of feeling more energetic and improving your health. Ultimately, you will feel proud of yourself for being your own best health advocate. If I can do this, so can you!

Following simple steps, together we will make shifts in your self-care, uncover your personal mind-body connection to health, and enhance your glow. Chronic inflammation is the devil! It is the catalyst behind many diseases including cancer, heart disease, diabetes, Alzheimer's and autoimmune diseases. Fortunately, by addressing the root causes of inflammation we can undo its damage and potentially reverse a diagnosis. Disease and dysfunction don't just happen. When we experience strange symptoms, we can thank our bodies for alerting us that inflammation is at work. Then it's up to us to heed the call and put our bodies back in balance before the inflammation progresses to dangerous diseases.

Think of the changes you will be making as a beginning of a very enlightening journey of learning, nurturing, and healing. Who promised that we could always eat and behave the way we did when we were teenagers? Change is a constant we can count on! And we can rely on ourselves to nourish our minds and bodies with attentive self-care, restoring us back to balance. With the Food-Mood Method, you will take care of your body, and your mind will thank you. You'll take care of your mind and receive the benefit of a balanced body. Self-care will be your ticket to symptom-free, medicine-free, vibrant health.

This process of transformation requires faith in yourself, recognizing that the old ways of doing things, your old habits, are no longer working for you. This change can only happen if you are truly willing to take yourself on! Just the fact that you've picked up this book makes me think that you are. If you are teetering on the edge, maybe it will help you to know that, after a while, through dedication and consistency, the healthy changes you make will easily become part of your everyday life. Effort and struggle will fall away as results start to emerge. You will feel great, and what better incentive is that? So are you ready? Okay, then let's get cooking!

# Part One

CHAPTER 1

# My Wellness Adventure

I'd like to tell you more about my own personal experience with illness and healing in an effort to give you hope that you, too, will overcome whatever ails you. When I've shared my story with women in my community, many excitedly told me that it struck a familiar chord with them. As I share my journey here, perhaps it will resonate with you as well.

It's a chicken and egg kind of story. Did my "woe is me" outlook on life come before the gut permeability and inflammation, or was it the other way around? Maybe the sequence isn't as important as the big picture: Food and mood are intimately connected to wellness.

In my early thirties, my husband, Rob, and I moved from New York to the San Francisco Bay Area with our two small boys. We were on an adventure, and we had a deal. Rob would do research at the University of California, San Francisco for two years, and then we would return to New York where he would pursue a fellowship in plastic surgery. I put my life on hold, like so many dutiful wives, and followed my husband to support him and his career. During Rob's research stint, UCSF offered him a fellowship position. I knew how important this could be for my husband's career, so I gritted my teeth and agreed to stay for another two years. However, once again, at the end of the fellowship, UCSF offered him a job. Hospitals in New York City had no openings, so how could he refuse?

During these years, although I was saying "yes" out loud, I was silently screaming "no!" And I was getting resentful. I had left all of my friends and family back East, and I still didn't feel rooted or comfortable yet in California. I was practically raising my kids alone, and was working part time to help support us. I began to see the world through the eyes of a victim. With few outlets, I took my anger out on my husband, and our marriage began to suffer.

Meanwhile, during this five- or six-year period, a very painful and unattractive new development cropped up on my back: cystic acne. Boils, as they are referred to in the Bible, are one of the ten plagues! It seemed like a punishment from above. In reality, the condition was the first sign of an internal imbalance. I was prescribed an antibiotic, and, as directed by my doctor, stayed on it for several *years*. That's a very long time considering antibiotics kill, not just the bacteria doing harm, but the good bacteria in the digestive system too.

Soon after, I also began to notice strange new symptoms: chronic pain in the largest thumb joints; aching muscles between my shoulder blades; a numb pinkie toe; brain fog; and a persistent, dull sore throat. Inflammation was taking its toll. For these symptoms, I went to a rheumatologist who determined I had six out of the eleven symptoms and blood markers for the auto-immune disease lupus. What a terrifying diagnosis! As shocked and frightened as I was, my husband, with his in-depth medical knowledge about lupus, was even more so. My doctor offered me a steroid, the only treatment option at the time. But from some-where deep inside of me came a hunch and hope that I could find a better solution. I rejected the steroid and set out on an Internet journey of discovery, steeping myself in information about inflam-mation and autoimmune diseases.

Thank goodness for the web. What I learned after months of reading reliable medical studies and scientific articles were these important facts:

- My symptoms were all manifestations of an overactive immune system that was causing inflammation in my joints, muscles, and nerves.
- Autoimmune diseases are the result of a perfect storm of three components: first genetics; second an environ-mental trigger such as a food, toxin, trauma, or infection; and third leaky gut syndrome (a permeable digestive lining).
- A leaky gut allows partially digested food to pass through into the bloodstream. There, the body perceives it as a harmful pathogen and attacks it as it would attack any foreign invader such as bacteria or a virus.

## Time for a Personal Inventory

Wait a minute. Was I in the middle of the autoimmune perfect storm? I began taking stock. First, did I have a gene for autoimmunity? I thought about my late mother who had had hypothyroidism. Every evening her muscles ached. I also discovered that several of my aunts and grandparents had rheumatoid arthritis and hypothyroidism. It seemed likely that I could have the genes predisposing me to an autoimmune disease. Looking at the health of your immediate and extended family is a good jumping off point for piecing together the root causes of your own symptoms. Ask yourself the same question I asked myself. Does anyone in your family suffer from an autoimmune disease?

Next, I thought about what environmental triggers I may have been exposed to. A toxin, a problematic food, an infection, or my long-term antibiotic use perhaps? Then I learned something that really amazed me: Environmental triggers can actually influence genes, turning them on or off and affecting everything from the metabolism and one's energy to the progression or prevention of diseases.[1] Oddly, even emotional stress and physical trauma can act like environmental triggers, creating genetic changes. And, then, this blew me away. The act of giving birth can have the same traumatic impact on our genes as, say, a car accident. In fact, my doctor mentioned that autoimmune diseases are especially prevalent in women who have had two children. Who knew?

Further, I learned that food intolerances play a role in inflammation and autoimmune disease, each often associated with specific symptoms. Gluten (found in grains such as wheat, rye and barley) is often the food trigger at work. Certain proteins in gluten can help cause a permeable gut, which then allows them to mischievously pass through the membrane into the bloodstream. This causes a confused response from our immune system—the bodyguard that ambushes destructive visitors—inciting our anti-bodies to (correctly) attack the gluten and (incorrectly) assault our healthy tissues. This can lead our organs to malfunction and joints, muscles, and nerves to become inflamed. For example, gluten is often the culprit behind the immune system's attack on the thyroid gland, causing the autoimmune disease Hashimoto's thyroiditis, the most common form of hypothyroidism. Surprisingly, the gluten protein gliadin actually resembles thyroid tissue. Curious to see if my hunch that gluten was wreaking havoc with my own thyroid gland was right, I asked my primary care physician for a blood test, and guess what? I had Hashimoto's, too. I must have had a leaky gut—but why?

Fast forward a decade and I now know the most common causes of leaky gut, which include:

- Viruses, bacteria, and protozoa
- NSAIDs – non-steroidal anti-inflammatory drugs such as ibuprofen and aspirin
- Gluten intolerance and other food sensitivities
- Depleted oxygen supply to the digestive system, which can occur during surgery or shock
- Glyphosate – a chemical herbicide heavily used on genetically modified (GMO) crops[2, 3]
- Cytotoxic cancer drugs[4]

With so many risk factors around, it's a miracle our guts are ever intact!

## First Step: Detoxing Body and Pantry

What's a woman with autoimmune symptoms to do? Starting with the most likely food trigger, I made the commitment to ditch gluten for several months, the length of time recommended for detecting a change in symptoms. With the support of a friend who has celiac disease—a hypersensitivity to gluten in the small intestine—I learned some simple substitutes for gluten-rich breads, desserts, grains, and condiments. Coincidentally, two more friends were also suffering from joint and stomach pain, skin blisters, and swollen fingers, and were ready to try a gluten-free diet. We certainly were a motley crew determined to find natural solutions to our odd symptoms. This was eight years ago when gluten sensitivity was not yet well understood, so I was lucky to have the support of friends, helpfully sharing this experience as well as ideas for healthful gluten-free cooking.

Frustrated at the two-month mark when I didn't feel relief, and in the face of much skepticism, I persisted, determined to complete the experiment. My young boys were embarrassed when I'd ask waiters if my order contained any gluten. Some family and friends, particularly on the East Coast, were dubious of a gluten remedy, thinking this must be some new California trend. However, sure enough, after three months, all of my symptoms disappeared! When I went back to my rheumatologist, he was just as surprised as I was that all of my lupus blood markers were gone as well. I had discovered my own food trigger through a food elimination trial and was on my way to becoming healthier and more energetic than, well, maybe ever. And, a decade later and still gluten-free, while I continue to have the presence of Hashimoto's thyroiditis antibodies, I have never needed thyroid medication. Is it a coincidence that in the 10 years since my journey began, gluten has received widespread attention due to the relief many people feel without it?

With my health improved and a new habit of label reading, I began to wonder what else I was eating and cooking that might not be serving me or my family well. Though I knew enough not to take my kids to McDonalds, I have to admit, I succumbed to buying lots of convenient, packaged foods to make cooking quicker, lunches easier to pack for school, and my little boys happier (or so I thought). Think Lunchables, Bagel Bites, Pizza Pockets! The food industry "had me at hello" with their intentionally enticing ads, promise of ease and happy families, and addictive sugar-filled products. Those are powerful forces tricking us into mindless spending and eating. And they make eating highly flavored yet nutritionally empty foods a difficult habit to break.

Because I had to read ingredient lists to steer clear of gluten, I started to notice how many unpronounceable chemicals and preservatives there are in processed, packaged foods. Remember seeing the effects of the last major oil spill, the ducks and gulls struggling under the mess of black crude? I began feeling like one of those sweet birds only burdened with processed food. This sludge is harmful, and I needed to get it off me (and my family)!

Going gluten-free was the impetus I needed to begin phase two of my food makeover: eat clean— that is, consume food in its whole, natural state, not processed, refined, or adulterated; add tons of veggies and fruits to my diet; and steer clear of chemicals, pesticides, dyes, added sugar, hormones, and antibiotics. The more I learned about the connection between food, inflammation, and disease, the more vigilant I became. Was it any surprise that my boys had all sorts of food-related, inflammatory issues including eczema as babies, chronic diarrhea, IBS, an ADD diagnosis, and cystic acne? Finally, I woke up!

Cleaning out a pantry filled with sugary cereals, cookies, pancake mix, breads, nut butters, pudding and gelatin mixes, as well as industrialized canned soups, packaged dinner "helpers," mac and cheese, sauces, chips, crackers, and processed lunch meats, I became an unpopular mom for a while. What, no Doritos? Let's face it; we all want to make our kids happy. But by switching to organic foods to avoid artificial junk, pesticides, and herbicide-rich GMOs, and making whole foods such as fresh vegetables, scratch-cooked eggs and oatmeal, homemade soups, grass-fed meats, fish, stew, and chili, plus whole grains such as rice, quinoa, and brown rice pasta, I began to see that food's connection to health was much larger than just gluten. My boys' acne and diarrhea was gone. I could have kicked myself for feeding them all that junk for so long! In addition, my husband lost over 50 unwanted pounds (along with the help of a new exercise routine) and felt more energetic, optimistic, and confident than he had in years. And my energy, skin, and sleep kept improving. With such benefits, incorporating these changes became easier and easier.

I know now that there are other bonuses, too. A healthy, anti-inflammatory diet free of foods that trigger reactions can provide mental health benefits, stronger hair and nails, and long-term disease prevention. The bottom line? Diet can improve health and even reverse disease. Don't just take my word for it. Many people have healed their debilitating autoimmune conditions, diabetes, and cardiovascular disease with changes in diet. You'll read some of their stories peppered throughout this book, reinforcing the idea that food changes can heal such conditions as celiac, Sjogren's, Raynaud's, and assorted skin maladies. For more inspiration, I encourage you to do further research on diet's impact on health. Learn how Terry Wahls, MD, reversed her debilitating MS symptoms with a healthful diet. (http://terrywahls.com) And check out many compelling stories in documentaries like *Forks Over Knives*; *Fat, Sick, and Nearly Dead*; and *Food Matters*.

Happily, the "inconvenience" of healthful cooking from scratch inspired a new way of life for my family. The mouth-watering aromas and sounds of sautéed onions, bubbling soups, and roasting chicken are the signs of home and sharing time together. I let my gourmet mother, the Food Network, cookbooks, and blog recipes inspire me, then I tweak the instructions when necessary to avoid inflammation-triggering ingredients, creating my own healthy and satisfying recipes (see Chapter 7).

With some time and practice I have become a passionate cook and have taught my boys to cook, too, empowering them to be stakeholders in their own health. For fun, we invented a competitive cook-off modeled after the show *Throwdown with Bobby Flay*. We choose a dish—a pasta, taco, or even a sandwich—and we each make our own version with a personal, signature twist. A designated judge does the taste testing and proclaims one "chef" the winner. We love this stimulating, healthful, and helpful family time. The guys have become great cooks themselves, helping me in the kitchen, and translating those skills to college, where they have taught their peers about good nutrition.

This journey has been satisfying and informative, and I am wiser and more joyful than I've been in decades. Does any of this ring a bell for you? Are you wondering whether your symptoms may be inherited and related to food and toxins? Are you getting excited to do your own food diagnostic and makeover? Can you imagine your whole family benefitting?

## Second Step: Detoxing The Mind

*We are shaped by our thoughts; we become what we think. When the mind is pure, joy follows like a shadow that never leaves.*
- Buddha

At the same time that I was renovating my diet, I needed to address the anger and stress I was still feeling. This was no way to live my life and, quite possibly, could have undone all the good my new way of eating was doing. The mind is inextricably connected to the health of the body and can contribute to the root cause of diseases. Stress makes us more susceptible to infectious pathogens and changes the behavior of our genes. While I loved being a mom and appreciated the Bay Area's fresh, flavor-packed food, the focus on fitness, the breathtaking landscapes, hummingbirds, and rainbows—treasures not visible through New York City skyscrapers—I was still unhappy and angry that we had moved to California. Missing New York and the comfort of old friends and family, I began to take it out on my husband. Have you ever lashed out at someone you love only to wonder what the heck has gotten into you? The poor guy was working crazy hours, building a career as a surgeon, and taking care of women with cancer. What he needed most was a positive home as a refuge.

Instead, I was on autopilot, unconsciously and unconstructively demeaning him for everything from his gaining weight to the way he chewed! Needless to say, our marriage was suffering. I couldn't seem to shake the negativity and mistakenly thought I required the positive energy of others to lift me up and fill my cup, a dependence that left me feeling powerless. What I didn't yet know was that what I needed all along was within me. A positive spirit with a large dose of gratitude would be the key to more loving connections with others, the perspective to create something new in my life, and a vastly improved mood.

Years of sadness made me realize I needed to take action. "Snap out of it!" I told myself and, suddenly, something made me listen. In hindsight, it's clear that this adversity was my opportunity for growth and change. Thankfully, I love exploring the unconscious mind with various therapeutic modalities. I believe that by shining a light on the issues that keep us stuck, we learn about ourselves and find freedom to choose a different path. That notion led me to try a weekend-long transformational coaching workshop I'd heard about. Seriously? *Girl from New York moves west and attends "new age" transformational event while throwing back wheatgrass shots and kale chips!* Can you feel the skepticism that almost prevented me from enrolling? Nervous but curious, I went with the intention of finding more joy and abundance in my life. On day one, the coach was talking about having gratitude for our miraculous lives. Convinced he didn't know me and therefore couldn't be speaking about my life, I stood up in front of 150 people and asked, "How do you know if you have a good life?"

"Are you homeless?" he replied.

With his simple answer and a crowd of supportive witnesses, something shifted in me. I suddenly understood that the way we feel about life comes from our personal perspective, and that's something we get to choose. To elucidate, Nelson Mandela, a great example of steadfast optimism and belief in his vision, chose this perspective even under the most dire and difficult of situations. While imprisoned, lonely, and often sick from damp conditions, he wrote a best-selling book on social justice and oppression, and ultimately, influenced the transition to a democratic South Africa. Even in jail, he focused on the possibility of making a difference in the lives of others rather than feeling victimized or powerless.

That weekend was the beginning of what was to be a remarkable, life-changing experience. Taking responsibility for my perspective about everything in my life left me feeling strong and grateful, able to make a change. With excitement and newfound access to the love I always had for my husband, I raced home to apologize to him for demeaning him over the years in California. Since I no longer needed to play the victim, our marriage grew stronger and even our conflicts, once complicated and loud, became easy to resolve. Interestingly, as I learned that weekend, conflicts are the result of one person wanting to be right and make the other person wrong. They are generated by beliefs we develop when we were young, often brought about by traumas we experienced from our interactions with peers, parents, and other adults in our lives. Negative beliefs stem from unconscious feelings of unworthiness or defensiveness and, if left unresolved, can trigger distress and the urge to battle with people. Like gluten and poor nutritional choices, these beliefs and subsequent conflicts put stress on the body and cause inflammation. To undo this unconscious reaction and heal from our past traumas, it can take significant work through coaching, therapy, positive psychology, or meditation, all of which raise our awareness and heal our self-sabotaging emotions.

Can you guess what happened to that cup half-full? I filled it up. Since then, yoga, meditation, and therapy have enabled me to become even more aware of the critical voices in my head, and to consciously look for the best in myself and in others. In psychology, this is called "reframing." In my life, I call it a godsend.

## The Curse Becomes a Blessing

Was my autoimmune condition a horrible diagnosis or an inspiring journey? In place of victimization and anger, I now feel responsibility, gratitude, and calm; my marriage thrives; my relationships are stronger; and I love living in the Bay Area. I also still have some times of sadness and worry. Who doesn't? But I now appreciate that these emotions, just like joy, creativity, connection, and love, are part of the miraculous sensations of being alive.

Feeling relief motivated me to stick with my new food habits and, because I felt happier, to try other healing self-care rituals. Yoga, meditation, running, green smoothies, and more laughter became a part of my daily agenda. Taking one small step toward improved health became a daily breath of fresh air! That's key. The secret to making a lifestyle shift is taking small steps and finding support. Want the ticket to a life filled with joy? Practice gratitude, heal sabotaging beliefs, and deliberately look for the best in others. More on these practices ahead.

### DEACON'S STORY

I was a typical kid, born in the 1970's in England. I grew into my girth around the age of nine, when my parents decided to open a Toys & Sweets shop. I used the confections to help soothe the verbal wounds about my weight that school bullies administered to me on a daily basis. During a school weigh-in, I was berated by the administration for being so unhealthy. They suggested I follow a school-approved diet. The diet literature highlighted how "bad" it was to be fat, and that it was not only unhealthy, but also unsightly. Needless to say, their disapproval and judgmental comments—"corpulence is a disease"—

intimidated me. Though I tried the new diet, I also consumed more chocolate, and by the time my family immigrated to the U.S. in 1987, I topped the scales at 270 pounds. I was 14 years old.

Now in the New World, I had a new identity! However, by the second week of my new school, when the novelty of my accent had worn off, kids started to bully me again because of my weight. And, with the quantity of food one could purchase cheaply in the U.S., much of it poor quality processed foods high in sugar, I went from 270 to 320 pounds over the course of 18 months. In addition, I developed asthma and a serious case of eczema. I couldn't ride my bike for long because I would start to wheeze, and in the summer, the sweat of any activity would cause my skin to flare up. For my skin disorders, I saw dermatologists who prescribed awful topical treatments. For my asthma, I went to pulmonologists who gave me prescriptions for various inhalers. I also had countless blood tests to determine what was wrong with me. But none of the medicine I was given ever really helped me overcome what was at the root of the problem: a simple addiction to sweets and processed food, developed as a way to soothe the stress of being bullied.

Fortunately, in 1988, I met a woman who completely changed my life. She took me to an Ayurvedic clinic in Massachusetts to have an evaluation. Ayurveda is a 5,000 year-old practice from India aimed at balancing the body through proper diet and lifestyle. Yoga is part of this same system. The doctor there told me I had a serious imbalance in Pitta and Kapha, two of the three Ayurvedic "doshas" or body types. An imbalance of Pitta meant that I had a lot of inflammation, as exhibited by my asthma and eczema. My Kapha imbalance showed up as weight gain and lethargy. In Ayurveda, it's easy to determine symptoms by looking at qualities of the elements on which the doshas are based. Vata, for example, is comprised of space and air. Vata imbalances cause issues of mobility, dryness, and scattered thinking. Pitta (fire and water) causes excessive heat, inflammation, and short temper when imbalanced. Kapha (water and earth) imbalances produce issues of sluggishness, weight gain, and emotional turbulence.

The Ayurvedic physician gave me a comprehensive briefing about my body and its inherent ability to go out of balance based on what I was eating, thinking, and doing. I received a complete food guide about what was right for my body and what would cause me challenges. Stress was also a factor in my imbalances, so I learned Transcendental Meditation and a simple yoga practice. Never once did the doctor say the word "diet" in the context of losing weight. Rather, he felt that if I simply reduced and removed the foods he considered to be inflammatory, my body would be able to recalibrate itself, and therefore help me heal. Ayurveda has a saying: " When food is of poor quality, medicine is of no use. When food is of good quality, medicine is of no need."

His advice was simple: start slowly and gradually add in new practices to reduce the need for sweets. It worked! Though the first two months were a little rocky, over the two years that I followed his plan I went from 330 pounds with asthma and eczema to 170 pounds with clear skin and no breathing challenges. I had reprogrammed how I dealt with stress, no longer reaching for sweet treats and adopting new, healthier habits.

Ayurveda made me realize that our bodies have the natural ability to heal themselves, as long as we understand what our symptoms are "telling" us. The practice points out that each of us is completely individual. With our unique physiologies, we need to examine whether we are consuming foods that may heal us or harm us. Our states of balance and stress, as well as how certain foods affect us, directly correlate to our overall health and wellbeing.

For over 26 years, I've been able to maintain my weight, my health and my stress levels through the practices of Ayurveda and yoga. It was simply logical, and once I understood how the foods I was eating affected me, I was able to make a shift in my approach to my health.

## CHAPTER 2

# Love Yourself Enough to Make Change Possible

*Eating well is a form of self-respect.*

-David Avocado Wolf

Now that you have had a glimpse into the possibility of improving your health naturally, do you feel you are worth the effort? You are! Your presence on this planet is important. Your life has value, and the rest of us are counting on you to love yourself enough to treat yourself well, to be your best self. Healing one person at a time is how we heal the world. Let's start with you.

Real, lasting change does not come from a diet book or a new fitness craze. How many times have you thought about getting healthy? What about the number of resolutions you have made and diets you have tried only to end up slipping back to where you started? Sustainable change comes from deliberate choice followed by long-term repeated action. You can accomplish this! Every effort-filled moment of work you put into your goal amounts to greater certainty of eventual success. Any new behavior—including a hobby, career, or skill—takes time and effort to master. Nothing comes to you without some work. But on the other side of this work is the ability to feel proud of yourself and to own your own health.

I'll be honest: Dark chocolate is my weakness. So is binge-watching TV. Pair the two together, and I find myself mired in a mindless trap, opting for a moment of pleasure that only leads to an unconscious pattern of overdoing and regret. Even writing about it here has me becoming more attuned to my potential for self-sabotage. It takes work to break my habit. One day at a time, with awareness and intention, I rotate between various substitutes (sweet potatoes, fruit, granola, and coconut milk) to satisfy my sweet tooth so that now this once nightly habit has become an occasional indulgence. But I could easily slip into that routine again without a conscious effort to make a difference in my blood sugar, my weight, and my energy.

## Change is Good

Change can be a hard-fought struggle. It can seem overwhelming to think about a new way of behaving. Adopting new actions and learning why they are beneficial can feel like work. It takes mental energy. But change leads to growth and strength. Think about it. What change have you undertaken that has made you stronger? How did you feel after making it? What did you lose during the process? What did you gain? If transformation feels challenging to you, I'd like to propose a new perspective on change, one that is fun and creative. And one that is all about the very best self-care. It can be exciting to buy a new jacket or shoes because these items breathe new life into your view of yourself. Believe it or not, incorporating healthier eating and new habits into your routine can have the same effect. It gives you a fresh, inspiring point of view about your body and your identity as a beautiful, healthful human being. Plus, healthful eating is the most basic form of self-care.

Even without my own personal experience of finding relief for joint pain and muscle aches and feeling alive and well again, it's hard to ignore the strong evidence that suggests natural healing occurs through improvements in self-care. Scientific research even shows that food and mood make an impact on disease at the level of our genes (more on this in Chapter 5).

Gaining knowledge and awareness of what both science and anecdotal evidence indicate about achieving good health is the first step toward change. The old saying, "What I don't know won't hurt me" just isn't so. With awareness comes choice. Combine that with encouragement and action and you've got a recipe that will make a difference in your life.

## Self-Care is Born from Self-Love

It took me almost 40 years and an autoimmune diagnosis to realize that my health is important, and that I am worth the attention, time, and money it takes to be healthy. So are you. Self-care is a form of self-love. And that is quite different than being selfish.

Setting boundaries for yourself can be challenging. We've gotten praise our whole lives for sacrificing, helping others, putting ourselves last. That behavior has its place. But when was the last time you got a pat on the back for putting yourself first? Probably never, but I urge you to adopt the conviction that you are worth spending time and effort on and to develop a clarity of purpose: What do you most want in your life? How do you want to feel? I love the airline safety analogy, "Put the oxygen mask on yourself first and then on your children." Truly, if you are not taking care of you, you cannot possibly offer others your best self. To garner support for the dietary and lifestyle changes you are about to make, tell family and friends you are taking care of yourself so you can be there for them when they need you.

And then there's the thought of spending on ourselves. Do you balk at paying a few extra dollars for organics each week, but shell out $600 for your cell phone or shoes? Aren't you more valuable than these things? When I realized this odd discrepancy in my own life, it occurred to me that spending a bit more for organic and healthful food whenever possible is a smart investment in my health. Be imaginative. Think of the ways you'll save money when you eliminate the afternoon sweets, Starbucks coffee drinks, acne products, weight loss diets, and so on.

## Courage and Clarity

The thought of change can be difficult, if not overwhelming. We all know there are things we can do to improve our health, but we avoid them. Why do we do that? I know I could get out more often in nature with my dog and with friends. Fear—fear that it will take too much time from my busy day, that I won't enjoy it, that it won't make any difference in my outlook or health—gets in my way. Other times, I just want to eat what I want to eat and do what I want to do without restrictions. Can you relate? What does it take to change and adopt new, healthier behaviors? It takes a clear vision of what you hope to find on the other side. It takes some faith in health, in yourself, and in change. If the old way isn't working, what have you got to lose?

## CLARIFY YOUR GOALS AND INTENTIONS

There must have been something that drew you to this book. What do you hope to gain by understanding food and mood and by experiencing the Food-Mood Method? Take a little time to think through and get clear about your goals. On a sheet of paper, write out the answers to the following questions.

1. At what point in your life did you feel your best?
2. During that time, what was it that had you feeling your best?
3. What are your top three health goals now? Examples: pain relief, more energy, better sleep, more joy.
4. On a scale of 1 to 10, 10 being most important, rank the three goals you just created.
5. Anything you marked with a 7 or above in question #4 is very important to you; what's been getting in the way of achieving these important goals?
6. Why are your goals important to you? Get very specific. Examples: I'll be a good example of health to my family; a promotion will be possible; I'll spend more time having fun with friends.

7.   What is the cost of not making these changes?
8.   What do I need to let go of to make these changes?
9.   What do I intend to learn from the Food-Mood Method?
10.  Who or what can I count on for support?

Once you are clear about why you are about to undertake the Food-Mood Method, keep these intentions very present in your mind. You may want to post your answers to the above question-naire on a wall, fridge, or mirror where you can see them as a reminder. It may seem easier to keep things *status quo* than to make the effort. It may seem daunting to tackle a change—where will you find the time, the money, the ability to remember everything you have to do? However, once you finally commit and incorpo-rate a new behavior into your daily life, it becomes a "no-brainer," like brushing your teeth. Thought is no longer needed as the new behavior becomes automatic. And once you are on the other side of your symptoms, it's easy to stay there—it's a self-perpetuating feedback loop of feel-good actions!

## Finding Support

For many of us, it's very difficult to change our behavior alone. The positive support of a partner can make all the difference, encouraging us and keeping us accountable for our new actions. However, not everyone feels the same way about support, and it's important to know what works best for you. Do you do better in partnership, sharing the experience, and having an external source of motivation? Or do you work best alone, preferring to hold yourself to account and depending on your own internal drive for incentive? If it's the former, reach out to a coach, friend, or find an accountability partner as you proceed on your health quest. As an integrative health coach, I help my clients get very clear about their health goals, and together, we devise a plan that will help them succeed, one step at a time. (To work with me and to sign up for my monthly health tips and recipes, visit www.nanfosterhealth.com.) Whether or not you work with someone one-on-one or an accountability partner, consider joining community events such as workshops, classes and sporting clubs (running or biking groups and marathon trainings, for example), which offer excellent change-making structure and support.

There are also spontaneous reinforcements that may come up naturally as you proceed through the Food-Mood Method. Positive changes provide great psychological benefits. Imagine finding out that a particular food is causing you acne, asthma, pain, fatigue, or even diabetes, lupus or cancer. Would that be enough of an impetus to change your eating behavior and remove the offending food? How about tasting the true essence of a food for the first time? I know that ditching processed and sugary foods for scratch-cooked meals changed my taste buds. Suddenly, the flavor of real food, even vegetables, seemed incredibly delicious, while packaged foods tasted like chemicals. Talk about a no-brainer! It became easy to change.

# Release Self-Doubt to Access Self-Reliance

*Don't believe everything you think.*

- Jim Collins

Whether you reach out to others for support or go it alone during the Food-Mood Method—or for that matter, during any life quest—it takes internal conviction and self-reliance to make lasting changes. Low self-esteem and negative beliefs about ourselves can lead us to self-sabotage. Imagine a young woman standing alone at a party gazing at clusters of people engaged in animated conversation. She knows no one and often feels out of place in social settings. She is three feet from the nearest group, and her body is shyly turned away from them as she looks down at her hands. She wants to connect, however, no one comes to talk with her, and she doesn't join any conversations. Glancing at her, the others get the impression that she wants to be alone or feels anti-social. Her self-doubt and body language create a circumstance of aloneness even though she wants to be noticed. Now, imagine instead that she has the intention of meeting people, and despite her anxiety, turns towards the nearest group, makes eye contact, and introduces herself, taking responsibility for her own connections. She becomes engaged in conversation.

Many of us frequently believe that other people are better, funnier, and smarter than us, and that we are not good enough to be successful or happy. Many of us also believe that external forces determine our success or happiness, and that the way we feel is due to our circumstances. I used to feel that way, a lot. And guess what I found out? The mind often lies. Did you know that eyewitness identifications of supposed criminals during police lineups are wrong 75 percent of the time? Research shows that inaccuracies rise with length of time from the crime and other corrupting influences. The eyewitnesses, however, are convinced that their memory is correct, flawless. Our thoughts and beliefs actually help *cause* circumstances. In turn, that confirms how we feel. It's like a feedback loop or a self-fulfilling prophecy. And, frankly, our limiting beliefs are a lot of BS! You and I were born with everything we need to create the life we want.

To feel emboldened and find self-efficacy, we must first break free from the deep-seated stories we tell ourselves. Stories are core beliefs developed in childhood that, in a negative vein, sound like "I'm not enough," "I'm unlovable," "I don't matter," or the more aggressive, "I'll show you." Do any of these resonate with you? Where do these stories come from? An event happens in childhood and our innocent minds, feeling sad and ashamed, make it mean something about us. Abuse and neglect may cause these perspectives. But even less traumatic events, including unsupportive comments or put-downs from parents, teachers, and peers, can cause us to perceive that we are bad, wrong, and unworthy. As adults, these false beliefs can make us defensive or upset, causing conflict. Ever witness someone get furious or self-righteous and have no idea why? It's likely stemming from an unconscious story about themselves.

We all experience this phenomenon. Stories are a source of your judgment of yourself and others. However, you can build awareness of your attitudes and where they come from. And with awareness, these stories lose their grip, though they may always be present. Your mental health depends on how you think. It is time to stand in the truth of who you really are. You are wonderful and amazing!

## DISCOVER YOUR STORY EXERCISE

Take a moment and see if you can find your story. See if you can recall your earliest memory of someone hurting you.

1.  What's your earliest traumatic memory? Close your eyes to think back and remember.
2.  What did you feel in that moment? Where do you feel it now in your body when you recall that memory? Chest, stomach, shoulders?
3.  What did you decide about yourself in that moment years ago?
4.  How long have you been telling yourself this story?
5.  What is the impact of your story on your life today?
6.  Can you forgive yourself and others involved? Forgiveness doesn't condone the people involved; it just helps us move past what happened.
7.  Can you move past what happened or will you let other people's actions keep you stuck in the past?
8.  Think of a personal strength. Close your eyes and recall a time using that strength. Where do you feel this memory in your body?
9.  Choose a new positive story to replace your negative belief such as "I am good," or "I am brave."
10. Practice replacing your old story with your new one often. Share it with people close to you. Through understanding,

compassion and acceptance, you can surrender your stories and secrets and move past these false perceptions.

11. Seek the help of a therapist or use the Emotional Freedom Technique (EFT) to help free you from stories. (See Resources, page 198.)

Freedom is a choice. It is time to reclaim yourself. There is nothing wrong with you. Nothing has ever been wrong with you. Remind yourself of this every day and tell yourself, "Nothing and no one has the power to take away who I came here to be."

I discovered my own story through enlightening discussions and exercises at transformational workshops, in coaching training, through yoga and meditation, in therapy, and by talking with family and friends. I vividly remembered a moment in my life when I decided, "I'm not good enough." At age eight, I had a Halloween party. After collecting our loot, we returned to my family's apartment for dessert—special witch hat ice cream cones. A bossy friend blamed me for something she had done, and my mom, overhearing this, sent me straight to my room with no dessert. In that moment I decided I wasn't worth as much as the friends who were joyfully eating ice cream just outside my door. My friend had lied. My mother had neglected to discuss it with me and chose to punish me at my own party. And I hadn't stood up for myself. For over 30 years, I unconsciously held that belief. With work to reveal my story, I forgave my friend, my mother and myself for the parts each of us played in that scenario. Now, I am very aware when this perspective comes creeping in. Because it is so much a part of my consciousness and not my unconscious mind, I can tell myself "No, that's a story," and it vanishes.

## HANNAH'S STORY

As a kid, I had frequent constipation. There were weeks when I was only able to go to the bathroom a couple of times. My mom, other family members, and some friends, had similar problems. I never thought much of it. Then I got older and had the opposite problem; in college I tended to get diarrhea. Additionally, I've had frequent yeast infections throughout my life.

Other symptoms were mounting evidence of a bigger issue. As a kid, my ears and feet would get uncomfortably hot and itchy, turn purple, and blister when exposed to the sun. My feet became worse in the winter or if I left my socks on too long. Finally, I got my first diagnosis from a dermatologist who biopsied one of the blisters on my toe: perniosis, an inflammatory condition typically seen in cold and damp conditions. A topical ointment was prescribed.

Next, I developed severely dry eyes. I started wearing contact lenses in sixth grade and soon thereafter my eyes became dry and irritated. They'd often get infected, too. Doctors told me that my eyes were very sensitive to even the slightest bit of bacteria and recommended the most moisturizing type of daily lenses. My eye dryness, though, only became more severe over the years, and I had to significantly limit the time I was wearing lenses, or I developed capillary scarring. In college, I mostly wore glasses.

Lastly, in high school I noticed that it sometimes took me longer to study or complete assignments than my peers. For this, I was prescribed ADHD medication. Since my mother had several autoimmune diseases, she suspected a bigger issue might be celiac disease. With her urging, I went to see a rheumatologist and had blood work done. It came back positive for celiac, Raynaud's, Hashimoto's thyroiditis and Sjogren's syndrome. Finally, I had my answers. Not surprisingly, several autoimmune conditions run in my family.

Among the many recommendations my rheumatologist made, not eating gluten made the biggest difference in my life. It completely changed my digestion, which is normal now. I had no idea that I was experiencing fatigue before (tired was just normal for me), but it was clear after becoming gluten-free that I was because I now have much more energy and less of a "foggy" brain. I'm still taking my ADHD medicine, but I am now on the lowest dose. I think being gluten-free has also helped my eyes a bit. Though they are still very dry, and I can't wear contacts for many days out of the week, I can wear them for longer hours. Hot eye compresses and drinking a ton of water have been helping too. My extremities are okay with the Raynaud's. I kind of just live with it and try to keep my hands and feet warm. I don't have blistering or rashes anymore.

Initially, when I was in college, it was really difficult to go off gluten. It was hard to stop drinking beer and eating all the gluten-filled things in the dining hall. Ultimately, experimenting with living gluten-free and listening to my mom, who said that I needed to stop for at least a month to really experience any changes, was what it took for me to change. When I actually got to the one-, then two-month mark, I really noticed a big difference. Occasionally, I would slip up and have a piece of pizza or whatnot, but that's what really made me realize that gluten affected me so much. It just wasn't worth it to have those things. While I have felt better being gluten-free for the past four years, recent blood tests showed that my blood markers are relatively the same. I actually had to start taking a small dose of thyroid medication several months ago.

I think that people who experience a lot of digestive problems and fatigue should seriously consider getting tested for autoimmune disease. Going off gluten is really not that difficult in the long run. There are tons of alternatives and substitutes for basically everything that you want with gluten. Additionally, restaurants have tons of options and have gotten a lot better at being educated about celiac disease.

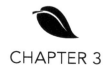

CHAPTER 3

# You Are What You Eat and What You Think

*Soul and body, I suggest, react sympathetically upon each other.*
-Aristotle

L ike a successful team in any sport, our bodies win when each "player" is playing its part well. An assist from a healthy diet and positive thoughts help with digestion, nutrient absorption, cellular function, and hormone balancing. In turn, when these conditions are optimal, we receive a boost in immunity, mood, and outlook. A bad day for any player can cause other team members—including the brain, skin, liver, joints, and thyroid—to play poorly. The antidote is to address the whole team at once (like a good coach does) through both food and mood. And balance is the name of the game.

Okay enough with the sports metaphors. What throws us off balance? Stress.

Believe it or not, scientists now know that thoughts, feelings, and food can influence the behavior of our genes as well as the nature of our day.[5] Positive thoughts and a good quality diet result in healthier gene behavior while negative thinking and poor quality eating have the ability to cause disease as a result of the stress they induce. While we typically think of stress as something that stems from anxiety—things like work demands, family illness, a loved one's death, and moving—the body also experiences stress from poor diet, nutrient deficiency, toxins, and some medications. Negative emotions and beliefs impart stress as well.

Throughout this book, I use the term "stress" to refer to an impact from any source that causes the body to become imbalanced. While life throws us many curveballs, and we cannot control all the stressors we experience, many diseases are preventable and reversible by fixing imbalances in food and mood. By putting the body back in balance, we give it the opportunity to heal itself, which is its inherent natural tendency.

## A Gut Reaction to Stress

Let's start with stress' effect on the gut microbiome, which plays a critical role in helping us fight germs. (The microbiome, you will remember, is the combination of good and bad bacteria in the gut.) Scientists now understand that the microbiome contains 100 trillion bacteria. That's ten times the number of human cells in our bodies! In a healthy gut, the bacteria help digest food, boost immunity, and make mood-elevating neurotransmitters like serotonin. A healthy microbiome depends on the diversity and balance of good to bad bacteria. Normally, 85 percent of the bacteria are helpful bugs while 15 percent are the bullies waiting to pick on the good kids.

Trying to preserve this balance for health is a lifelong endeavor as the microbiome is fragile and easily disrupted. Helped along by any one of life's stressors, the bad bacteria can flourish putting us into an imbalance called gut dysbiosis. Under this condition, many diseases and unhealthy conditions can be ignited, among them weight gain, diabetes, depression and other mental health disorders, heart disease, cancer, and autoimmune diseases. It can even accelerate aging. Fortunately, gut dysbiosis typically gives us clues in the form of physical symptoms, such as systemic inflammation, pain, muscle aches, gastric reflux, diarrhea, gas, bloating, as well as mental health symptoms like anxiety, depression, and hyperactivity.[6] The good news is that, if we pay attention to these issues and attend to them by reducing or eliminating the stressors, we can head off the imbalance before it leads to more serious problems.

In addition to causing gut issues, chronic stress can cause hormone imbalances. A constant toxic overload increases production of the stress hormones cortisol and adrenaline, causing the release of triglycerides and fatty acids, which can increase bad LDL cholesterol over time. And, because hormones are closely interconnected, these stress hormones cause imbalances in other hormones, such as insulin, estrogen, and testosterone. Those imbalances, in turn, can suppress or overstimulate the immune system, putting us at risk of illness and disease. Further, hormones and the digestive system are a closely-knit team. Have you ever had gastrointestinal distress during menstruation when hormones are changing? When one system is affected, the other is likely reacting, too.

To make matters even more interesting and complex, what we eat affects how we think and feel, and what we think affects how we behave, what we crave, and how we eat. Whew! The term "you are what you eat" is more accurate than one might imagine. The food we eat literally becomes our blood, our cells and our tissues. It affects hormone balance, protein production, immunity, inflammation and, ultimately, our thoughts and moods. As such, food is more than just sustenance; it is spiritual.

What it basically comes down to is this: Balance is what we seek; stress in its many forms is what we loathe; beautiful, healthful food is what we need to heal. And when we view our multi-faceted system as an integrated whole, we are left with the most basic recipe for wellness: Reduce our toxic stressors to bring the body and mind into balance, tamp inflammation, calm the immune system, and prevent disease. Easier said than done? When we have knowledge and maybe the help of others, the task is simplified and rewarding.

## WHAT DOES AN INTEGRATIVE NUTRITION HEALTH COACH DO?

If you're new to the idea of Integrative Nutrition®, you might wonder what an IN health coach does. Let me fill you in. As I work with clients, I consider the health of the whole person as well as their lifestyle. What is the state of the person's "primary food" intake, and by that I mean what is the food that nourishes their souls: relationships, careers, physical fitness, and spirituality? Those things are as important to overall health as "secondary food," i.e., the food we eat. The importance of both primary and secondary foods to a balanced, healthy body and mind cannot be overstated. What the coaching process does is help shine a light on behaviors in each of these areas that might be getting in the way of a client's health goals.

Each client's first step in his or her personal food-mood makeover is to ask for help. That alone is an acknowledgement of one's self-worth! Over time, as I build trust, listen, and ask key questions of my clients, coaching sheds light on their habitual stress-inducing behaviors. This awareness enables clients to make slow, steady changes. Here are a few examples of the types of issues I see in my practice (all names that follow have been changed):

- Jeannie's goal is to sleep through the night. Through Q&A and discussion, we realize she consumes candy bars and her third coffee every afternoon at three o'clock to get through the workday. She walks to her job, but hasn't begun an exercise or meditation practice to revitalize and de-stress. Thus, the cycle of exhaustion persists.
- Wendy feels stressed out, and her digestive health suffers. She and Bill argue often. Wendy is feeling unloved and unseen in her relationship, and her stress is manifested as stomachaches

and diarrhea. Before she can heal, Wendy needs to address the underlying emotions and behaviors causing her illness.

- Ellen has gained weight and struggles with frequent headaches and food cravings, which she often feeds with chips or a bagel. She drinks several glasses of wine each night at restaurants and bars with friends or at home alone. Dehydration and sugar highs and lows from wine and refined carbs are keeping her in a vicious cycle of weight gain and sugar addiction.

By building awareness of the food and mood contributors to stress, we unlock the pattern of behavior in which my clients have gotten stuck. After we've zeroed in on what needs to change, I help them adopt the healthy habits that support wellness, including exercising, drinking more water, substituting nutrient-dense foods and satisfying beverage alternatives for empty-calorie snacks and drinks, nurturing more supportive relationships, and creating positive sleep environments.

## Diet and Disease: A History

*"What an extraordinary achievement for a civilization: to have developed the one diet that reliably makes its people sick!"*

- Michael Pollan

We can put a man on the moon, but we can't solve the American diet crisis? Where did we go wrong? Looking at the current state of American health, how startling is it that we are in the midst of the worst health crisis this nation has ever seen, with rates of obesity and diabetes at all-time highs and heart disease and cancer rates climbing?[7,8] Or that, with billions of dollars spent on research, the U.S. is still number 28 on the list of 34 free-market countries for life expectancy? That this is the first time it is predicted that life expectancy will shorten during our children's lifetimes? And that, while we are currently living longer than we were several decades ago, 70 percent of us are on medication to manage the symptoms of chronic diseases and ailments that we now know can be treated and even reversed through proper nutrition and exercise? As Americans age, we rely on doctors to manage diseases sometimes for decades. In fact, a 2011 study determined that we are living fewer *healthy* years than we did a generation ago.[9] The bottom line: A sedentary lifestyle, toxin exposure, and the typical American diet help fuel inflammation and diseases.

Unfortunately, it's likely that the food you've been brought up on is the root cause of feeling unwell, gaining weight, and developing diseases. In fact, the Standard American Diet (SAD), followed by many as a result of a faulty scientific study in the 1950's mistakenly suggesting we would minimize heart disease on a high-carb, low-fat diet, has turned out to be a disaster. This tragic recommendation led to dangerous dietary shifts, welcoming an onslaught of "low-fat," processed, and fast foods high in refined carbohydrates and sugar to the market. Ironically, these are the very foods that are a major cause of obesity, hypertension, high cholesterol, heart disease, cancer, diabetes, Alzheimer's, and depression.

The truth, as we now know, is that healthy fats protect us from these ailments. Sugar, on the other hand, whether it comes in the form of table sugar, soda, fruit juice, or refined carbs like bread, bagels, pasta, pretzels, and baked desserts, causes system-wide inflammation and destruction. Ultimately that leads to an increase in fat storage, plaque formation, and a brittleness in our vascular system, which can:

- set the stage for heart attacks and strokes;
- cause blood sugar highs and lows throughout the day that can increase anxiety, cause hormone imbalances, cravings, fatigue, and acne;
- feed the bad bacteria and yeast in our guts.

And sugar is as addictive as heroin and cocaine!

Adding insult to injury, the food industry has infused their products with highly inflammatory polyunsaturated and trans fats, chemicals, additives, herbicides, and pesticides. Antibiotics turn up in our meat, and endocrine disruptors such as bisphenol-A (BPA), PCBs, and phthalates line the plastics and cans that hold our food, seeping into what we ingest. The U.S. Food and Drug Administration has even admitted that a typical American consumes 50 pounds of chemicals from food each year. Our wholesome ancestral way of eating is virtually gone, taking our good health with it.

Even with our current understanding of these problems, there is still steady action working to maintain the *status quo*. We are inundated with advertisements, convenience foods, fast foods, and ingredients that are good for business, but bad for health. Pharmaceutical, processed food, and health insurance companies work hard to meet and exceed their bottom line; they're hungry for profit and, as a result, uninterested in research into natural healing.

As I've noted, I'm married to a doctor whose work I respect completely. Yet that doesn't change the fact that conventional medical schools have also overlooked natural healing and nutrition. And they are only beginning to teach the importance of the microbiome. Now that it is cutting-edge science, it's hard to ignore! While doctors play a critical life-saving role in surgeries, grave illnesses, and mental health crises, they are not likely to search for or treat the underlying cause of disease. Instead, physicians are taught to ameliorate chronic conditions with prescription medicines.

How familiar we are with the quip, "Take two of these and call me in the morning!" And while prescription medicines will serve to quell symptoms—they can lower cholesterol, thin the blood, kill bacteria, balance blood sugar, lessen pain—they don't reverse disease and often have serious side effects that can cause new problems. Antibiotics, for example, can nudge the microbiome off balance in favor of the bad bacteria. Diabetes medications keep Type 2 diabetics dependent on medicine to regulate blood sugar, but don't resolve the cause of their metabolic syndrome. Non-steroidal anti-inflammatories (NSAIDs) such as ibuprofen can cause a leaky gut as well as heart disease. This is where diet and lifestyle changes can make an enormous difference, treating the root cause of these conditions and often precluding the need for medication.

One of the other problems I see with traditional medicine is that doctors are taught to regard the body as separate parts and systems. You see a cardiologist for your heart, a hematologist for your blood, a rheumatologist for autoimmune diseases, and so on. That can have benefits in certain cases, but it also leads to doctors missing the big picture: the integrated whole. The truth is, we are not the sum of many parts. We are an interconnected system, each part of which relies on the others and thrives when conditions are balanced. With medical school curricula practically devoid of nutrition education as well as the self-interests of the food, pharmaceutical, and medical insurance industries dominating what's available to the average person, we must learn to be the best caretakers of our *own* health.

## A Paradigm Shift

Ironically, while 70 percent of Americans are currently on medication, nature has been there all along offering her natural remedies. Did you know that a mostly plant-based diet can stabilize blood sugar and build immunity; that herbs detoxify the liver; that spices can prevent cancer and reverse inflammation? Fortunately, because of recent research and findings about the benefits of good nutrition—and thanks to books, articles, and lectures from key pioneers, including doctors (Jeffrey Bland, MD, Andrew Weil, MD, Mark Hyman, MD, Daniel Amen, MD, David Katz, MD, and Frank Lipman, MD to name a few), as well as naturopaths, health coaches, nutritionists, epigeneticists, and activists—natural approaches are beginning to catch on. Our health paradigm is finally shifting. We now know that healthy habits can actually prevent and reverse many chronic diseases. To sum up, here's what prevention and longevity require:

- Real food, not boxed or processed
- A mostly plant-based diet with healthful fats and proteins
- Low to no refined carbs and sugar
- A multicolored array of veggies, fruits, herbs, and spices
- Organic foods to eliminate dangerous chemicals
- The removal of food triggers
- Calming strategies such as exercise, meditation, and connecting with others
- A positive mindset

The body does its best on our behalf, striving for homeostasis and filtering out toxins in its natural quest for health. Let's show it some love so it can perform at its best. It is up to each of us to become informed, act as our own health advocates, and strive for a healthy mind and body with a plant-based whole food diet and healthful, mood-boosting life practices. One person at a time, we can create a ripple effect, changing the health of this country.

Amazingly, recent discoveries in the field of epigenetics show that a healthful diet, lifestyle, and mood can actually prevent the 90 percent of diseases that are genetically predetermined. We can literally change the course of our health by what we put in our bodies because food and lifestyle change the expression of our genes. Isn't that remarkable? We are not stuck in a particular genetic destiny. Food and lifestyle can influence what was once thought to be inevitable! (See Chapter 5 for more on epigenetics.)

This phenomenon is illustrated best in regions where people live the longest, healthiest lives on the planet. Called "Blue Zones" and studied by National Geographic fellow Dan Buettner, these five regions (including Sardinia in Italy; Ikaria in Greece; Loma Linda, California; Okinawa in Japan; and Nicoya in Costa Rica) have the largest populations of centenarians—more than 10 times that of other countries. And these folks are active, hiking, gardening, playing, and chopping wood even at 102! What's their secret? They reduce stress naturally with a great attitude and a lifestyle that centers on a plant-based diet; consume limited amounts of meat; cook from scratch; move often; put family and loved ones first; have social connections; incorporate spirituality into their lives; take naps; have hobbies; relax; and have a purpose in life. We can learn a lot from these happy, engaged, unmedicated, and symptom-free elders.

It's possible to cultivate that lifestyle even here in the U.S., beginning with the Food-Mood Method. Not only does it translate into a healthy, vibrant, engaged life, but knowing you can count on yourself for your own best care and happiness is powerful and uplifting stuff too.

## More on Mood and Wellness

*Your mind is in every cell of your body.*
-Candace Pert, PhD

Like food toxins, emotional stressors such as chronic anger, loneliness, anxiety, shame, overwhelm, and sadness have an impact beyond the brain, changing the microbiome, lowering immunity, and triggering illness. Research has discovered that such emotions cause inflammation and diseases.[10,11] But I didn't need science to tell me that; I could see it in my own home. With looming deadlines and pressure to succeed, my boys always got colds and viruses right before finals in high school. On the other hand, no member of my family ever gets sick on vacation. We are more susceptible to infection when life amps up the stress. In fact, research on the microbiome and on cell receptors inside the gut reveals a synergistic relationship between the gut and the brain. Interestingly, this connection may be the reason we have a "gut feeling" about something and why both physiological and emotional forces can create fierce internal disruption. If you are experiencing pain, depression, anxiety, ADHD, weakness, low energy, brain fog, skin outbreaks, and even stubborn weight gain, it is important to unravel the mysteries of your own potential gut-brain/food-mood sensitivities.

Further, our emotions are linked to immunity in several complex ways. According to pioneering neuroscientist Candace Pert, Ph.D. whose research focuses on the biochemistry behind psychology, "...neuropeptides and their receptors are the substrates of the emotions, and they are in constant communication with the immune system, the mechanism through which health and disease are created."[11] With regard to neuropeptides and disease, Dr. Pert's work supports well-documented scientific findings about the connection between emotions and heart attacks. For example, research has shown that heart attacks and death rates are highest on Monday mornings, the days following Christmas (among Christians), and right after Chinese New Year (among Chinese)—that is, on days with a strong correlation to emotions.[11]

It is believed that the immune system responds to negative emotions by releasing certain peptides (compounds in the body made up of amino acids) that cause plaque formation in the arteries. Conversely, happy emotions seem to have a protective effect on the immune system. Happiness, put under the microscope, reveals the release of the health-protective neuropeptide norepinephrine. Norepinephrine binds to the cell receptors that also happen to bind to the cold virus. The more norepinephrine, the fewer receptors available for the virus, thus the fewer colds. Our immune system seems to protect us best when we are at our happiest.

Given that the mind has the power to heal or harm the body, what is your state of mind right now? Like my scheduled gym workouts, I've made comedy and sweet Internet animal videos mandatory mind exercises. Research shows that our happy hormones flow when our brain experiences love, connection, and humor. And it's so much better for you than sugar!

In another area of research on both the placebo effect and the Pavlovian response, scientists have also determined an irrefutable connection between mental conditioning and physiological responses. In both cases, the mind-body response to a drug or placebo paired with a stimulus—the sound of a bell or a sweet taste—conditions the body to respond to the stimulus. Later, even when the drug or placebo are removed, the stimulus continues to elicit the effect. The power of the mind is amazing!

## DEBBIE'S STORY

Fifteen years ago, I was diagnosed with an autoimmune disease called pemphigus vulgaris, a condition that causes blisters or sores on the skin or mucous membranes. In my case, it was painful lesions in my mouth and a variety of other places on my body. I didn't realize then what it would mean to have a chronic autoimmune condition: a regimen of daily steroid medications and their side effects, a susceptibility to other illnesses, and unexpected flare-ups. I also developed intestinal problems within a few years of being diagnosed with and taking medication for my pemphigus.

With time and the help of a nurturing and knowledgeable nutritionist and health coach, I learned how to understand my body and its needs. While I stayed on the medication, I adapted my diet according to my body's sensitivities—and it saved me! Eating fewer carbs and avoiding gluten and dairy altogether meant less cramping and more energy; more raw fruits and veggies reduced heartburn; and avoiding sugar helped me feel healthier overall. I no longer had to live my life feeling like I had a chronic case of the stomach flu, and by removing the physical stress of feeling sick all the time, I have also been able to keep my pemphigus quiet.

My friends often tell me that they are surprised by my self-discipline. I explain to them that it's not a matter of discipline when dietary changes allow me to feel comfortable and help me keep my autoimmune condition in remission. It's my best-case scenario.

## CHAPTER 4

# Immune Systems Gone Wild: Inflammation and Autoimmune Disease

*All disease begins in the gut.*

- Aristotle

U nder normal circumstances, the immune system is brilliant. It rushes to attack invaders such as bacteria, viruses, and toxins. And the inflammation, swelling, and redness it causes in response to those invaders is appropriate; it actually keeps us healthy. The immune system also remembers the invaders so that next time they try to sneak in, wham, the attack is fast and furious. Normally, immune attacks are acute responses that occur as needed. And, normally, the immune system should mimic the Goldilocks protocol: not too hot, not too cold, just right, producing the perfect inflammatory response.

All too commonly, however, we are over inflamed. How does this happen? One reason is that, because most of our immunity resides in the gut, by bombarding ourselves with processed junk foods and toxins, we confuse the immune system's natural process. And when the influx of junk and toxins is chronic, the immune system can become overactive creating inflammation in joints, muscles, nerves, blood vessels, and organs, and leading to disease. Picture the crazy, whirling Tasmanian devil leaving a trail of destruction in its wake!

Chronic toxin exposure can switch the immune system from bodyguard to enemy, instigating an attack on our own tissues and making us vulnerable to food allergies and intolerances, autoimmune diseases, and conditions commonly associated with aging such as heart disease, cancer, and Alzheimer's. In fact, arterial plaques—deposits that cause the number one killer, heart disease—are thought to be the body's way of patching vessel walls that have been damaged by inflammation. It is estimated that 75 percent of us have food sensitivities, a detrimental (if not quite allergic) inflammatory reaction to certain foods.[12] If ignored, food intolerances (a term used interchangeably with food sensitivities) can add fuel to the fire, causing even more inflammation. Yet whether inflammation produces obvious sensations such as pain and stiffness, or stealth and silent symptoms as it does in cardio-vascular disease, there are actions we can take to minimize our disease risks.

## INFLAMMATION TRIGGERS

- Chemicals
- Pesticides
- Herbicides
- GMOs
- Food Intolerances
- Preservatives
- Growth Hormone
- Food Dyes
- Antibiotics
- Sugar
- Emotional Stressors
- Excessive Physical Exertion
- Gut Dysbiosis

# Food Allergies Versus Intolerances

We are each bio-individuals—one person's food may be another person's poison. While my husband thoroughly enjoys his morning coffee, my heart palpitates and my tongue gets numb even with a few sips. Typically due to the absence of a digestive enzyme, a *food intolerance* can cause inflammation-related symptoms in the digestive system such as gas, bloating, acid reflux, and diarrhea as well as skin issues, anxiety, headaches, and joint pain. It can also cause a drop in the feel-good neurotransmitter serotonin, negatively impacting mood and cravings. A *food allergy*, on the other hand, typically causes a response in the immune system. And while an allergy is often associated with rashes, hives, itching, and shortness of breath, it can also cause many of the same digestive problems as food intolerances. Unlike the obvious food allergies requiring immediate attention (think children's nut allergies and EpiPens), an intolerance can be more subtle, and it often takes two to three days for the body to react. This delayed response is why it can be difficult to understand a direct cause-and-effect between the food and the symptom.

Over time, a food intolerance left unheeded causes inflammation in the gut, putting us at risk for even more food intolerances and for autoimmune diseases. By eating foods we are intolerant to, we may unknowingly trigger a negative chain of events, including an immune system response. Antibodies are produced against what is perceived as a dangerous invader, and inflammation occurs throughout the body. Food triggers will frequently keep the immune system in overdrive by continually stoking the inflammatory response.[12] And the immune response can progress into autoimmune diseases while we unwittingly continue eating the culprit.

The good news is that by identifying and removing your food trigger (or triggers), you can eliminate your symptoms, improve your health and your mood, and even banish cravings. Therefore, your first step is to learn what to eat and what to avoid. It takes some trial and error to determine if you can tolerate a particular food. By becoming your own forensic nutritionist through food elimination in the Food-Mood Method, you may discover the source of your symptoms. There are also tests available that can help you determine a food allergy or intolerance. Once you discover your triggers, you'll want to avoid them while you clean up your diet and replenish healthy bacteria in your gut. You may even be able to tolerate the offending foods (or food) once your gut is back in balance.

Interestingly, in some cases nature has provided us with a clue: The very thing we crave upon waking can be what we are sensitive to. What do you crave first thing? I used to crave coffee and bagels. No surprise that I cannot tolerate coffee and that gluten was responsible for triggering my autoimmune disease. Gluten is the most common food linked to autoimmune diseases. Dairy can also be a problem for some autoimmune conditions such as Hashimoto's thyroiditis. Other common food triggers include corn, soy, yeast, eggs, and, less commonly, citrus and nightshade vegetables.

How do we become food-sensitive? Many of us are born with inherited allergies and intolerances, and others develop them. Over time we can even develop a sensitivity to a food we've toler- ated well for years. Exposure to toxins, medications, and proteins within foods can trigger a reaction. Without knowing we have a food intolerance, however, we may mistakenly attribute diagnoses and symptoms to IBS, aging, depression, or menopause, and our doctors may reinforce these ideas. However, simply removing a food trigger can put the body back in balance, quiet the immune system, and improve nutrient absorption, all of which may natu- rally eliminate symptoms and improve our health.

## Food Intolerance Testing

Food elimination is an excellent way to determine a food intoler- ance, but specialized labs can also test your blood for sensitivities.

(Meridian Labs and Cyrex Labs are two examples of labs that do this kind of testing.) A functional medicine practitioner (MDs and others who take an integrative system approach to determine root causes of illness), integrative physician, naturopath, or some gastroenterologists can prescribe the test. If you continue to suffer with diarrhea, bloating, or gas, or your stool has undigested food particles, your practitioner may want to rule out other issues that could account for the problem. These include digestive enzyme insufficiencies, parasites, an overgrowth of yeast or fungus, and small intestinal bacterial overgrowth (SIBO), which is an abundance of bacteria in the small intestine that is normally found in the colon. Whether you have a food intolerance or not, these symptoms typically indicate an imbalance that needs to be addressed. The trigger might be stress, too much sugar, poor diet, chemical and toxin exposure, all things that can be alleviated by the Food-Mood Method along with any physician-prescribed treatments.

## COMMON FOOD SENSITIVITIES AND THEIR SYMPTOMS

| Food | Common Symptoms |
|---|---|
| Gluten | Rash, brain fog, diarrhea, joint pain, mood |
| Dairy | Constipation, sinus, asthma |
| Soy | Rash, hives, eczema |
| Corn | Rash, hives |
| Yeast | Diarrhea, vomiting, joint pain, fatigue, mood |
| Eggs | Rash, hives |

# Autoimmune Diseases

Interestingly, autoimmune diseases are all variations on one theme: antibodies mistakenly attacking our own tissue. The type of autoimmune disease that ultimately manifests depends on the tissue under attack. For example, with lupus, facial skin cells, liver, and joints are often involved; with Sjogren's the saliva and tear glands come under attack; with MS it's the central nervous system; Hashimoto's thyroiditis and Graves' disease involve the thyroid gland; rosacea and psoriasis affect the skin; Type I diabetes involves the pancreas; and with Crohn's disease the gastrointestinal tract is at risk. There are nearly 100 autoimmune conditions. And because misery loves company, frequently more than one autoimmune disease occurs at a time. For an autoimmune disease to occur, a trifecta of conditions—an environmental trigger, intestinal permeability, and genetics—must be at work. Let me tell you more about each one.

## 1. ENVIRONMENTAL TRIGGERS

Beginning with a rapid rise in man-made chemicals over the last century, the world we live in has changed. The water we drink, the air we breathe, and the food we eat is riddled with toxins. While, thanks to medical discoveries, we are living longer in the U.S. than previous generations, we are at an all-time high for obesity, diabetes, cardiovascular diseases, and cancer. Compared to a generation ago, today's children are exposed to more pesticides,[14] sugar, and food additives; more antibiotics and hormones from conventionally farmed cattle and chickens; and more chemicals such as the endocrine disruptors found in plastic, shampoo, and fire retardants. And these children are the first generation predicted to have shorter life spans than their parents.

Meanwhile, rates of food allergies among children climbed 50 percent from 1997 to 2011, according to a recent study from the Centers for Disease Control and Prevention.[1] Please pay close attention to what I'm about to tell you: This time period coincides with the introduction of Roundup-ready GMO (genetically modified) crops, crops designed to withstand being heavily doused with Monsanto's glyphosate-rich herbicide, Roundup. Scientific studies have revealed a connection between glyphosate and gut dysbiosis, celiac disease, gluten intolerance, nutrient deficiency, and cancer![2, 3]

At times, the immune system becomes confused due to exposure to toxins in our environment. There are so many possible triggers, it's remarkable that the immune system ever works well! By minimizing our exposure to toxins, we can reestablish a healthy microbiome and reduce inflammation, making a difference in our own health and potentially, generations to come. How do we do this? First, we can take action to make a difference in our food system. As we refuse to consume the food industry's unhealthy, processed junk foods, and the drug industry's quick fix, side-effect riddled medications, we increase demand for healthier options, causing companies to make change. In fact, in the past couple of years, several food chains have stopped using GMO ingredients, food dyes, and excess sugar, and have introduced more organic and vegan options. More improvements are under way. Our smart choices are causing food businesses to make changes for the better. A definition of "smart choices"—and the way to minimize your exposure to toxins and promote healing—is this: Eat a clean, organic diet (see Chapter 5 on eating clean). Substitute traditional body and cleaning products with natural versions. Filter tap water to remove chlorine, fluoride, heavy metals, and pathogens. Limit exposure to antibiotics, non-steroidal anti-inflammatory drugs (NSAIDs), and acid blocking and proton-pump inhibitors. While these drugs treat digestive symptoms, they not only miss the underlying cause of the problem, they can create additional health issues including gut dysbiosis, nutritional malabsorption, and intestinal permeability.

I want to emphasize that there is no need to panic, or to discontinue vaccines or antibiotics when benefits to the individual and the population outweigh the risks.[15,16] Our bodies are able to detoxify when we treat them well. By exercising, omitting trigger foods, and eating an organic diet that is especially high in cruciferous vegetables (including broccoli, cauliflower, Brussels sprouts, cabbage, collard greens, bok choy, arugula, and radishes) as well as other sulfur-containing foods (onions, garlic, eggs, to name a few), many fresh herbs, and green tea, we can help our bodies purge the toxins and heal.[17]

## 2. INTESTINAL PERMEABILITY OR "LEAKY GUT"

The root cause of immune overstimulation is unique for each person. However, there is one thing all autoimmune diseases have in common, and it's something you won't typically hear from your doctor: intestinal permeability or "leaky gut." Picture TV commercials demonstrating weak, disintegrating paper towels. Got the image? Intestinal permeability is an abnormally porous gut lining. It enables partially digested food, bacteria, and toxins from within the gut to pass through the intestinal wall into the bloodstream. There they can trigger the immune system, stimulating food sensitivities, inflammation, and an autoimmune reaction.

Many people have leaky gut and aren't aware of it because it doesn't always come with gut symptoms. What causes it? Intestinal permeability can occur from contact with many of the environmental triggers previously discussed because of their effect on the gut bacteria balance. For example, antibiotics are often implicated in a gut dysbiosis and leaky gut because we are overexposed to them: Besides the antibiotic medicines we are prescribed for illness, we consume the antibiotics given to conventionally farmed animals when we eat their meat.

Similarly, the Monsanto Company's herbicide Roundup, which I mentioned earlier, is used on both conventional and genetically modified crops, and has been linked to imbalanced gut bacteria, leaky gut, celiac disease, and almost every illness associated with our American diet.[2,3] "Roundup-ready" genetically modified crops are designed to withstand very high levels of the herbicide, which contains the chemical glyphosate. Even minimal exposure to glyphosate has been implicated in leaky gut.[18]

Currently, there are nine genetically modified crops on the market including soy, corn, cotton, canola oil, sugar beets (a source of table sugar), zucchini, yellow squash, Hawaiian papaya, and alfalfa. To make matters worse, glyphosate is also sprayed on conventionally farmed non-GMO crops such as wheat and sweet potatoes. Further, while GMO corn (and cotton) may not be sprayed with glyphosate, they are engineered to produce their own insecticide called Bt-toxin. This toxin is also implicated in leaky gut, imbalanced gut bacteria, and poor digestion. Currently there is no transparency or labeling law governing GMO foods nor the use of glyphosate on any crops. How many GMO foods do you think you currently consume? To be certain you avoid these toxins, choose certified organic foods (organic also means non-GMO) as much as possible.

Commonly eaten foods that seem perfectly harmless can also be a cause of leaky gut if we are sensitive to them.[4,13] This is why it is so important to uncover our food intolerances. Gluten, as you may well know by now, is one of the foods that has been implicated in leaky gut. Gluten consumption increases production of a protein called zonulin, which researchers have connected to a leaky gut in people with autoimmune diseases.

Many of the symptoms of leaky gut—chronic diarrhea, bloating, gas, and gastroesophageal reflux, among them—may result in the common diagnosis of Inflammatory Bowel Syndrome (IBS) or Inflammatory Bowel Disease (IBD). These terms are general labels for an inflamed gut and many doctors leave it at that without addressing the complex causes of the disease process that may be occurring. As previously discussed, environmental exposure, intestinal permeability, and genetics, are frequently at work behind the IBS, IBD, and other autoimmune diseases. Some health care

providers, fortunately, will bear this in mind. A savvy gastroenterologist, a physician certified in functional medicine, an integrative
physician, or a naturopathic doctor may offer specific tests for
gut permeability if you have IBS, IBD, or autoimmune symptoms.

It is, for instance, possible to diagnose leaky gut with the
use of a special sugar challenge test, a test of gut bacterial DNA,
or a less direct blood test measuring IgG and IgA antibodies for
specific foods and gut bacteria.[2] There are, however, limitations
to testing. While endoscopy, an examination of the body using
a lighted, flexible tube, enables gastroenterologists to make a
visual diagnosis of celiac disease by viewing flattened microvilli
in the intestine, it doesn't provide a view of a porous, permeable
leaky gut. That's why the condition often goes unrecognized and
undiagnosed.

But even without a definitive diagnosis, there are several
healthful steps that you can take to help heal gut permeability and
reverse symptoms. Eat organic. Avoid NSAID drugs, alcohol, and
antibiotics unless medically necessary. See a doctor to get tested
for and treat parasites, *H. pylori* and other pathogenic bacteria,
fungus and excessive yeast, nutritional deficiencies, and heavy
metals, each of which can contribute to gut dysbiosis. The good
news about a leaky gut is that, with attention, diligence, and time,
it can be mended. With the Food-Mood Method, you will clean
up your diet, eliminate food triggers, and calm your mind, all of
which help to heal a leaky gut should you happen to have one.

## 3. GENETICS

Autoimmune diseases are hereditary. If you are uncertain about your genetic history, check with your extended family. Knowledge is power. It enables you to be your own best health care advocate. I myself had a known family history of autoimmune diseases. My grandfather and aunt had rheumatoid arthritis and my mother had hypothyroidism. As a result, I knew to ask my doctor for the anti-thyroid antibody test when I suspected my overwhelming fatigue was due to Hashimoto's thyroiditis. Sure enough, the test was positive for Hashimoto's.

Information gives you the opportunity to take action. Once I had my diagnosis, I did research on the web and learned there is a very strong connection between gluten and Hashimoto's thyroid-itis, as well as rheumatoid arthritis, celiac disease, and many other autoimmune diseases. After I removed gluten from my diet, I never looked back—my thyroid condition has been stable without any medications for the past ten years. I attribute that stability as well as the disappearance of all of my lupus symptoms and blood markers to changes in my lifestyle.

There is also more to the genetics story. Recent scientific research in the area of epigenetics, the study of gene expression, has discovered that it is possible to alter gene expression—the on-off switch of our genes—through diet and lifestyle, thereby directly impacting the onset or progression of 90 percent of genetically predetermined diseases.[19, 20] The changes I made had an impact on my genes, altering their expression and the resulting proteins they generate. Your genes do not control your destiny.

Make choices that change your genes for the better! (For more on epigenetics see Chapter 5.)

## ARDITH'S STORY

Throughout my youth, I experienced eczema and brain fog and felt sluggish and listless, especially after eating pizza and bread. Later on, during my first year of college, I got mono with severe joint inflammation and hepatitis. I slept all day and night, and lost 20 pounds in three weeks with no exercise. For years, I experienced yeast infections and many strep episodes, had pockets in my tonsils filled with pustules, and a dry sore throat. Looking back, all of this seems relevant to what happened next.

At age 37, my body really got my attention. My children and I got the flu. A week after our recovery, I woke up in severe pain with a high fever and very swollen joints, this time with a vascular rash that looked like black marker lines all over my body. I had multiple tests, and one came back positive: parvovirus, thought to be a trigger for autoimmune diseases. Those weird symptoms were due to "serum sickness," an autoimmune reaction that poisoned my blood.

Curious and intent on connecting the dots on a lifetime of mysterious symptoms, I went to the library (this was during the early days of the internet) to research these conditions. Armed with new knowledge, I requested tests from my doctor for rheumatoid arthritis (RA), Sjogren's syndrome, and Hashimoto's thyroiditis. All were positive! I was prescribed prednisone for six months. On the steroid, I felt more mobility, and both the swelling and venous rash diminished. However, I gained 30 pounds and had to nap four times a day. With my mood out of control—I was often feeling very depressed and unable to accomplish much—I felt I had no choice but to stay on the drug.

To lose the excess weight, I researched autoimmune diets and nutrition. I was already a gym rat and an early adopter of green smoothies before they were popular. But the most significant change I made was to go wheat and gluten free. This was 1998, and people really thought I was nuts! But I still couldn't lose the weight. After several unproductive visits to endocrinologists and rheumatologists— and receiving the invalidating advice, "Oh sweetie, all you middle aged women come in here and expect to go on meds to lose weight, when you should just be going to the gym and eating healthier!"—I needed a second opinion. Finally, I found an endocrinologist who gave me total T3 and free T3 thyroid tests, which some endocrinologists don't offer. Armed with new thyroid medication, I was immediately energetic and the pounds fell off.

Meanwhile, something amazing was taking place within my body that I discovered during a routine blood work-up. Within 12 months, all of my autoimmune blood markers had miraculously disappeared. Even the antibody to hepatitis I'd had since I was 18 was gone. My docs couldn't explain this. They are taught that once you have an autoimmune antibody, it will be permanent. So I was deemed an unexplained miracle. I proudly take credit for this result, having brought it about with my own nutritional choices. Unfortunately, based on decades of misdiagnoses and partial facts, I developed a distrust of the entire medical community.

My takeaway: Always do your own research. Be curious. Ask questions. Research nutritional options on reputable websites, then dig further by finding the medical journal studies and theses that are referenced in articles you read. Lastly, and perhaps most importantly, know that it is normal to feel alone going through this process, but that, in fact, what you're experiencing is very common. You deserve to be supported without damaging your own self-esteem or dreams for a healthy future.

CHAPTER 5

# Hijack your Genetic Destiny

*Your genome reacts to everything from sleep to emotions to stress to exercise to movement to breathing to food.*
– Deepak Chopra, MD

As a teenager in high school biology, I learned that we inherit our genetic traits from our parents, setting in stone everything from our hair texture, eye color, and height to our risk of disease. Genes were a determining factor over which we had no control. If someone had a disease that ran in their family, they should assume they were at the mercy of their heredity.

Fast-forward several decades, and it turns out our genes are not our destiny. The field of epigenetics, the study of gene expression I mentioned in the preceding chapter, has opened our eyes to the fact that we can actually influence the behavior of our genes and alter our health. Since the 1990's, following the discovery of the human genome, epigenetics has determined that, though our genes are hardwired, their expression is malleable. So, while our genes hold the instructions to build the proteins, hormones and everything else our bodies are made of, many factors, including diet, lifestyle, emotions, and environment, influence how those instructions play out. Everything from the food we eat to the rage we experience sends messages to our DNA, impacting every cell. Could this be why my lupus blood markers disappeared?

One way that changes in DNA occur is through a process called DNA methylation. DNA methylation is a technical term for the addition of a methyl group to the genes, which then acts as an on/off switch. When we digest nutritious foods such as vegetables, the nutrients are altered biochemically to become useful to our bodies. During this process, nutrients such as folic acid and B vitamins donate methyl groups which get added to DNA strands to help quiet genes and alter gene expression. Certain methylation can cause harmful effects which helps explain how toxins can influence genes.

The findings related to this on/off switch are exciting: Positive changes in our lifestyle are directly linked to the development or prevention of many diseases, including cancer, autoimmune diseases, neuropsychiatric disorders such as schizophrenia and mood disorders, autism, and Alzheimer's disease. Not only does the methylation process benefit healthful eaters, but the health of their unborn children is affected as well since the epigenetic changes are heritable. When we provide the body with a nurturing, positive, non-toxic environment, it returns the favor with the most favorable expression of its unique genetic code.

According to Deepak Chopra, MD, "Ninety five percent of genes linked to disorders act as an influence. They can sway one way or another, depending on other factors. Your biology doesn't spell your destiny. You have many choices because 'other factors' include a vast range of influences such as diet, exercise, stress management, and emotional events we take as everyday occurrences."[20] These findings underscore the important connection between our lifestyle choices and overall wellness. Affecting us at the level of our genes, our choices are our gateway to shaping our body and mind.

## Eat Clean to Reset Your Health

*Don't eat anything your great-grandmother wouldn't recognize as food.*
- Michael Pollan

*Let food be thy medicine, and medicine be thy food.*
- Hippocrates

I happen to love the trendy term "eat clean." It's a great visual, bringing to mind gorgeous, bright green leaves, big brown nuts, and healthy, happy animals. We are clean fanatics in the U.S., showering more than people in most other countries, crazy for our antibacterial products (with the unfortunate public health consequence of newly developed, resistant bacteria), and fastidious about our car washes. However, we've been slackers with our food hygiene. It's time to get back to our ancestors' way of eating beautiful, natural food. To reiterate, eating clean means consuming food in its whole, natural state, not processed, refined, or adulterated. Real, whole food sits on the plate much like it grows in the ground.

A clean, anti-inflammatory diet is important for anyone who wants to live a healthy life and reset their genetic destiny. For me, removing gluten was my wake up call toward better health and to understanding the connection between what we swallow and how we feel. One step leads to the next.

As you know, diet has a major impact on inflammation and disease; poor dietary choices cause stress on the body leading to hormone imbalance, gut dysbiosis, intestinal permeability, immune activation, and inflammation. So, it was a no-brainer that my next step was replacing the toxic ingredients in my family's meals with healthy alternatives. Who knew that eating clean would lead to so many tangible benefits? Improved immunity, satiety, and mood; increased energy and weight loss; stronger hair and nails; vibrant eyes and skin; improved sleep and mental health—it was a veritable smorgasbord of positive transformations.

## The Clean Alternative

How do you begin eating clean? Well, are you using artificial sweeteners? Throw them away! They are exactly what we've been talking about . . . artificial chemicals. Aside from being carcinogenic, they actually *cause* sugar cravings. How about apples that are conventionally grown (i.e., not organic)? They are number one on the "Dirty Dozen" list of foods that retain the most pesticides. Swap them for organic apples. Okay, good start. To further eat clean, scratch the junk and sugar from your diet and choose the freshest, most nutrient-dense, and organic foods you can afford. Visit farmers' markets if you are lucky enough to have them nearby; you'll be supporting farmers who grow crops and raise animals responsibly *and* bettering your own health at the same time. Buying what's in season and grown locally is the best way to get the most nutrients and help the environment. Shop at stores for fresh, organic produce, grass-fed meats and dairy, and organic beans, nuts, seeds, and grains. Fortunately these items are now widely available.

Eating clean also means eating a mostly plant-based diet loaded with vitamins, minerals, and phytonutrients such as anti-oxidants. More specifically, at each meal, fill half of your plate with vegetables and fruit. Divide the other half into one-quarter whole grains and one-quarter clean proteins such as pastured, grass-fed meats, chicken, eggs, dairy, or beans. Add in healthful fats like olive oil, coconut oil, nuts, seeds, avocado, and wild cold-water fish high in omega-3 fatty acids such as salmon and sardines. (See the Integrative Nutrition™ Plate for a visual on eating clean.) These choices ensure we get the macronutrients (proteins, fats, complex carbs) needed to keep us satisfied.

Think about it: You eat to survive. You consume food that makes you feel full. Why would you choose empty calories? Consider the nutrient density of your food. Which foods provide the biggest nutrient bang for the buck? (For help determining the answer to that question, see the ANDI–Aggregate Nutrient Density Index–https://www.drfuhrman.com.) By increasing your food awareness, reading labels, and learning how food is grown and raised, you will gain the ability to eat smart—that is, it will be easy to choose the most nutrient-dense, health-supportive nutrition on the planet. Get back to our ancestors' way of eating real, whole food—the original "farm-to-table." It's a vital way of life.

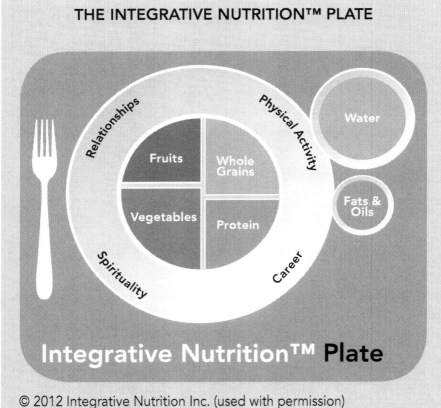

THE INTEGRATIVE NUTRITION™ PLATE

Integrative Nutrition™ Plate

© 2012 Integrative Nutrition Inc. (used with permission)
Based on the USDA "My Plate," the Integrative Nutrition™ Plate adds healthful fats, water and primary foods (our soul-nurturing lifestyle factors) to each meal.

# Tips for Wellness

You now have a wealth of knowledge about food and health. I hope you are inspired to tweak your own diet in pursuit of a symptom-free, vibrant life. A nutrient-dense diet providing vitamins, minerals, healthy fats, amino acids, and plant-based antioxidants helps your body and your brain cope better with stress, thereby helping you fight disease and maintain good health. Begin to read the labels in your pantry. Become a food detective. How many grams of sugar are in each item? Notice the many unpronounceable chemicals, preservatives, and additives. Keep in mind the hidden pesticides, herbicides, and added hormones, which you won't find on the label, but many of which are known carcinogens. The food industry is not on our side; it is all about their bottom line, not health and wellness. It's time to reclaim your health by cleaning up your act!

## DANIEL'S STORY

About 10 years ago, when I was 15, I began getting very bad, cramping stomachaches once a month. I was going to the bathroom only about every three days, and I felt uncomfortable. Other clues to my ultimate diagnosis of celiac disease were my halted growth and short stature at five feet tall in middle school, and, as my mother recalls often, wild, hyperactive behavior. My gastroenterologist confirmed celiac upon seeing the flattened villi in my intestine through endoscopy. I learned my stunted growth was due to an insufficient absorption of nutrients, and discovered that I had to give up gluten.

There is no one else in my family that we know of who has an autoimmune disease, and, back then, we didn't know how to go gluten-free. We relied on a family friend whose daughter has both celiac and diabetes. She essentially renovated our pantry, teaching my mother how to have a gluten-free household. My new diet helped me feel better, and I began growing again in high school. In college, I avoided the popular gluten-containing foods including pizza, beer, and bread. On the bright side, celiac helped me self-regulate my tendency to reach for baked sweets. And receiving a diagnosis gave me the ability to feel better and become healthy.

While going gluten free is much more popular now and celiac is a widely recognized disease, I recommend seeking an accurate diagnosis from your doctor to fully understand your symptoms.

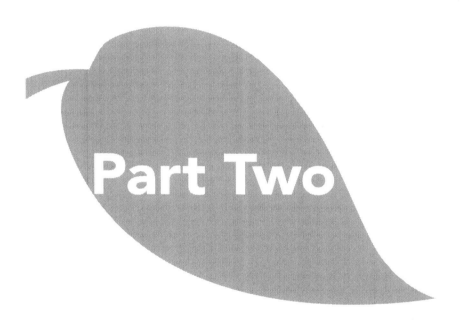

Part Two

CHAPTER 6

# The Food-Mood Method

My autoimmune diagnosis was the impetus I needed to become vigilant, to address my health, to nurture myself with self-care practices, and to create the Food-Mood Method. Now it's your turn! I'm so excited for you to discover healthy eating, learn whether you have a food intolerance and a leaky gut, resolve your symptoms, and reverse disease.

The Method is a six-step process of lifestyle practices that address body-mind wellness. I've included each of the healing actions that brought me enormous relief and have also provided practical exercises to help you incorporate those actions into your everyday life. This integrative approach will help you observe the cause and effect between your diet, your symptoms, and your mood. If your body is causing you discomfort, it's very likely a reaction to inflammation and imbalance. By balancing your gut microbiome and calming your mind, you can reduce the stressors that cause these issues and lead to disease. And by committing yourself to these practices, your body will thank you by naturally:

- Diminishing and eliminating aches, pains, tingling, and numbness
- Increasing energy
- Boosting nutrient absorption
- Relieving diarrhea, gas, bloating, and gastric reflux
- Strengthening immunity
- Protecting against disease
- Improving blood pressure, cholesterol levels, and cardio-vascular health
- Losing weight

Congratulations on committing to your own self-care and health!

# PART I. HEALING THROUGH FOOD

## STEP 1: RAISE YOUR SYMPTOM IQ

As you begin the Method, please work with your physician to arm yourself with information about your health. Even though the goal is to heal yourself by altering your diet and thought patterns, having the kind of tangible and measurable facts physicians supply will help you have a clear understanding of your baseline health. The key to healing is becoming very aware of what hurts and what heals you so you can create a personalized prescription for wellness. Use a fresh new notebook or pad of paper to answer questions and jot down notes. Writing down observations helps build mindfulness and provides a way to track your body's responses.

**FIRST: ILLUMINATE YOUR SYMPTOMS.**

In this Symptom IQ Exercise you will answer the following questions and record how you feel daily for seven days. Get clear on where and how the inflammatory issues are occurring inside your body. Use these notes when you visit your doctor to accurately report your symptoms.

1.  Each morning, upon waking, take a head-to-toe inventory of what ails you. Specifically, in what parts of your body are you experiencing aches, pains, tingling, tightness, and/or swelling?

2. On a scale of 1 to 10 with 1 being the least and 10 being the most, rate the aches, pains, and symptoms you feel in each area.

3. Twenty minutes to an hour after a meal, tune into your body again. Notice any changes and where in the body they are occurring. Write them down.

4. If you work out, keep your journal with you and note the type of exercise you did and whether your symptoms improved, worsened, or stayed the same.

**NEXT: WORK WITH YOUR DOCTORS.**

Taking a natural approach to healing and seeing doctors that practice conventional medicine don't have to be mutually exclusive. You can even take prescription medicine, if your symptoms demand it, and still use the Food-Mood Method to good effect, potentially improving symptoms naturally over time. Also, partnering with your doctors will help you understand what's happening inside your body by arming yourself with measurable lab tests and a diagnosis (or diagnoses as it is common to have more than one autoimmune condition at a time). Your primary care doctor is your symptom decoder and an insurance-covered visit to him or her is a good starting point. Your doctor can then determine what kind of specialist you may need to see. Here's what you should know before you go:

**Primary Care** Your doctor will likely do a complete blood panel and may want to check for C-reactive protein, a general marker of inflammation, which, best-case scenario, should be low. Note, however, that this test does not tell you what specific areas are inflamed.

Your doctor may also order IgG and IgA tests for food sensitivities. These are not very specific tests either (unless you have celiac disease) and may come back with false negatives, as they did for both of my sons and me. It takes specialized labs (such as Meridian and Cyrex Laboratories) to do more accurate food sensitivity blood testing. These tests are generally ordered through functional medicine, integrative, and naturopathic practitioners.

In addition, you can request blood tests to check your levels of vitamin D, magnesium, folate, and B12, which are deficient in many people and easy to supplement if necessary. Also ask whether testing your thyroid hormone levels and anti-thyroid antibodies (to determine if you have Hashimoto's thyroiditis) is called for.

**Specialization** Your primary care doctor may determine that you need to see a specialist. If your symptoms are mostly related to digestion, you will likely be referred to a gastroenterologist, who may check you for parasites, yeast, H. *pylori*, pancreatic enzymes, celiac disease, irritable bowel syndrome, ulcerative colitis, and Crohn's disease. If you suffer from joint, muscle, and nerve issues, you'll likely need a rheumatologist. That doctor will check you for autoimmune-related blood markers.

Once you have completed any blood tests, hopefully, you will be more informed than when you began. If you receive a diagnosis and/or a prescription for a steroid, a proton pump inhibitor, antacids, or ibuprofen, discuss the food elimination you are about to embark on with your doctor. It is usually best to stay away from these medications as they come with unfortunate side effects. However, if you are experiencing symptoms that feel unbearable, beginning on a regimen of medicine does not preclude your proceeding with a holistic approach as well. You can do both. The same is true if you are already on medication. Frequently people experience relief when they discover their own optimal food and exercise plan, enabling them to decrease or even eliminate their prescription medications.

**AND THEN: DO RESEARCH.**

Armed with this personal information about your symptoms—things like specific blood markers, indicators of inflammation, and a diagnosis—you now have the ability to do some homework. If you are curious about the underlying causes of your condition, use the Internet to find descriptive information. Conduct searches on your diagnosis, blood markers, and symptoms. But be very selective about which sites you read; there is a lot of misinformation on the web. Use only reputable sites such as those run by well-known research institutions conducting scientific studies, among them the Mayo Clinic, Memorial Sloan-Kettering, UCLA, University of California, San Francisco (UCSF), and the National Institutes of Health (NIH), or operated by well-respected natural practitioners

CHAPTER 6 PART I. HEALING THROUGH FOOD 99

such as Mark Hyman, MD, Andrew Weil, MD, Sara Gottfried, MD, Amy Myers, MD, and Dr. Joseph Mercola.

**LAST: CONSIDER ADDITIONAL PRACTITIONERS.**

For further support, consider the following types of practitioners:
- Functional medicine and integrative medicine practitioners –doctors who look at lifestyle factors to determine root causes, offer stool tests for parasites, yeast imbalance, SIBO (small intestinal bacterial overgrowth), as well as food sensitivity protocols
- Health coach
- Psychologist
- Acupuncturist and Chinese herbalist
- Ayurvedic practitioner
- Massage therapist

Now that you are becoming an expert on your own health, it's time to consider natural and alternative options. Continue to Step 2 of the Food-Mood Method to uncover any food sensitivities, and begin to detox and reset your body and mind.

# STEP 2: ELIMINATE FOOD TRIGGERS

You are about to embark on a detox that will help you discover food intolerances, remove the offending foods from your diet, and reset your gut. Grab your accountability partner(s) and tell them you are beginning the Food-Mood Method. Talk about your health goals (revisit the questionnaire on page 41) and the food elimination steps you are about to undertake. Will your partner take this journey with you, or just keep you accountable as you go? Day by day, meal by meal, step by step, your partner can provide you with positive reinforcement and validate your experience, while being honest and calling you out if you slip.

Imagine what life will be like without symptoms! Keep that image front and center. This is an exciting moment of discovery for you, and one that could lead to the health transformation you've been dreaming of.

**FIRST: DO A 21 DAY RESET.**

Remember, a food intolerance causes your immune system to mistake harmless food for a harmful invader and respond in the same way it would to a pathogen. By removing food triggers, inflammation is soothed, and the gut lining can heal. Gluten and dairy are most frequently the culprits behind inflammatory and autoimmune reactions, but other food sensitivities may be at work, too. A food elimination plan will uncover the offending foods. Choose a day to begin. What you will need:

- Calendar
- Journal
- Trigger-free foods
- Shopping lists, gluten-free guide, and recipes in Chapter 7

**To remove the common triggers of gut dysbiosis and inflammation, you will be eliminating gluten, dairy, corn, soy, and yeast for 21 days.** This is the length of time needed to allow your immune system to quiet down. It is easier than it may sound. Use the trigger-free shopping list and recipes in Chapter 7 to fuel your body with satisfying, healthful, delicious foods that support the best in you. You can do this!

Before you begin, remove temptations. Detox your pantry, fridge, and bar, clearing them of foods and drinks containing potential food triggers. Read labels. While you are at it, throw away or donate packages containing chemicals, preservatives, and other unpronounceable ingredients. *Beware of all processed foods, which can contain soy, corn, and gluten in forms that aren't always so obvious. For instance, many conventional chips and crackers contain GMO corn, chocolates contain GMO soy derivatives, and grains and flavorings contain gluten.* Purchase beautiful, real food in their place; using the gluten-free guide, shopping list, and recipes in Chapter 7 for ideas. If you have family members in your home who are not participating in the detox, create special areas for your detox foods to make it easier on yourself. Once your three weeks is up, you will add back each of the foods one at a time, as directed, except for gluten, which takes longer to elicit a response.

## A WORD ABOUT GLUTEN

If you have been diagnosed with an autoimmune condition, it's important to keep gluten out for good. If you have Hashimoto's or Graves' disease, it's imperative.[21] When gluten is a food trigger, it generally takes about one to three months to feel improvement after eliminating it from your diet. In rare cases, relief may be experienced within weeks. In some instances, people actually feel worse upon eliminating gluten. But this, in fact, is a sign that you may be gluten intolerant.

**During the reintroduction phase of the Method, gluten will not be reintroduced; keep it out of your diet for another three months to determine if you feel relief.** After 21 days, you will be much more comfortable with gluten-free eating. Lean on your accountability partner if necessary to keep you gluten-accountable. At that three-month point, you can then take stock of how you feel. And you may have indications before then. Trust me, if gluten is your trigger or you have an autoimmune disease, this is so worthwhile!

## A WORD ABOUT YEAST

Unless otherwise noted, baker's and brewer's yeasts and natural yeast can be found in baked goods (most of which also contain gluten), vinegar, aged cheese, fermented foods, and B vitamins.

## A WORD ABOUT CRAVINGS

The foods you crave may well be the ones you will have a sensitivity to, especially if you feel worse after eating them. Remember, when a food trigger is removed, typically cravings will subside, symptoms will disappear, and mood and health will improve.

**NEXT: ELIMINATE.**

For 21 days, eat what you want as long as it does not contain: **gluten, dairy, corn, soy, and yeast.**

**ALSO: KEEP A JOURNAL.**

During this time, note how food tastes and how your body responds. **Keep a detailed food journal, recording what you eat for breakfast, lunch, dinner and snacks for each of the 21 days.** (Don't forget, eating off someone else's plate counts). This will keep you accountable to yourself as well as very aware of what you are consuming. No cheating!

Sample elimination journal page:

|          | Mon | Tue | Wed | Thu | Fri | Sat | Sun |
|----------|-----|-----|-----|-----|-----|-----|-----|
| Breakfast |     |     |     |     |     |     |     |
| Lunch    |     |     |     |     |     |     |     |
| Snack(s) |     |     |     |     |     |     |     |
| Dinner   |     |     |     |     |     |     |     |

Sample reintroduction journal page:

|          | Mon | Tue | Wed | Thu | Fri | Sat | Sun | Notes |
|----------|-----|-----|-----|-----|-----|-----|-----|-------|
| Breakfast |     |     |     |     |     |     |     |       |
| Lunch    |     |     |     |     |     |     |     |       |
| Snack(s) |     |     |     |     |     |     |     |       |
| Dinner   |     |     |     |     |     |     |     |       |

## AND THEN: REINTRODUCE.

**At the end of 21 days, you will reintroduce each of the potential trigger foods, except gluten, one at a time, allowing three days before introducing the next one.** For example, reintroduce dairy on day 22, 23, and 24. Eat the food several times a day. Notice any symptoms including headaches, sinus, skin, and digestive issues, and mood changes. Record them in your journal. If you have a reaction, you should stop eating it. On day 25, 26, and 27, add organic corn, and then the organic soy on days 28, 29, and 30, keeping gluten out for another two months. (You're an expert on eating gluten-free now, so this shouldn't be terribly difficult.) Adverse effects during the three-day reintroductions are your clue to food intolerances. Remove the culprit and keep it out of your diet for another three months at which point you can try again to reintroduce it over a three-day period.

If the elimination has revealed which foods are your triggers, removing them is an enormous step in your quest for wellness. If you've added back these foods and have no adverse effects from any of them, it is safe to say that you are not sensitive to them. However, **if you still have symptoms, you can conduct this 21-day elimination process again this time eliminating eggs, nightshade vegetables (tomatoes, eggplant, potatoes, goji berries, peppers), nuts, and citrus.**

**LAST: HEAL.**

Experts suggest that the gut lining will heal after three months without food and other triggers. During that time, **research shows that it is important to replenish your gut with an abundance of different strains of healthy probiotic bacteria.** You can get that good bacteria by eating any of the following:

- Raw, fermented foods such as sauerkraut, kimchi, pickles, coconut kefir, and, if dairy isn't a trigger, dairy kefir
- Minimally washed organic plant-based foods[22]
- Prebiotic foods (those high in insoluble fiber that feed the healthy gut bacteria), which include artichokes, asparagus, dandelion greens, onions, garlic, leeks, chicory, blueberries, and bananas
- The amino acid glutamine, which is found in all animal protein, beans, cabbage, beets, spinach and parsley

You can also replenish the healthy bacteria in your gut by taking a variety of probiotic supplements. In addition, eat bitter foods such as dandelion greens, arugula, and olives to give your digestion some help by encouraging stomach acid secretions.[23] You can try reintroducing your food trigger again after those bacteria-restoring three months to see how your body responds. Except in the case of a gluten intolerance, a healed gut may enable you to tolerate the food again.

I hope you are feeling better already. And the effort you are making on your own behalf (and your family's) is inspiring. Keep up the good work! When eating out, continue to honor your body by asking for foods that are free of your trigger. Many restaurants are used to accommodating food intolerances, and if they're not, you can help them learn.

## STEP 3: EAT CLEAN. ADOPT AN ANTI-INFLAMMATORY DIET

*Eat food. Not too much. Mostly plants.*

- Michael Pollan

It's time to take the next step in your self-care. Just like a good shower, cleaning up your diet is refreshing and uplifting. Adopting a healthful, plant-based diet of whole foods is a way to reset your health and detox without deprivation. By following the dozen tips below and using the shopping list and recipes in this book, you will replace "dirty" foods–think processed foods, conventional crops, GMOs, and factory farmed animals–with clean, wholesome, and delicious choices–picture whole foods, organic crops, and pastured, grass-fed animals. Keep your food triggers out of your diet going forward. If you cook for members of your family who are not eager to clean up their diet, share your new foods slowly. As you begin to heal and have more energy, tell them what you are experiencing. Your enthusiasm will be contagious and your results inspiring.

**A DOZEN CLEAN EATING TIPS**

Many of the following tips also benefit the health of our environment. Together with the shopping guide and recipes, they'll help you be very clear and intentional about your healthful, new eating habits.

1. **Pantry reboot.** Remove temptations from your house. Can you imagine a drug addict attempting to beat addiction with drugs still in the house? Those Double Stuf Oreos? Out. Same goes for potato chips, traditional ice cream, and other unhealthy indulgences.

2. **Hydration.** Cravings and hunger are often actually due to thirst, so drink water (plain or with a squeeze of lemon) first thing in the morning and throughout the day. Consume half your weight in liquid ounces (e.g., 120 pounds = 60 ounces water). Caffeine-free herbal tea counts. Avoid sugary drinks including soda, fruit juice, and blended coffee drinks. Because alcohol and caffeine are dehydrating, limit alcohol to once a week, and consume coffee in moderation (1-2 cups per day). Notice if it improves your energy. I'm betting it will.

3. **Three meals.** To help keep blood sugar levels stable and avoid cravings throughout the day, eat three meals daily, starting with a healthful breakfast. Think lots of veggies, plus a clean protein and a healthy fat at every meal. If you get hungry between meals, choose a few healthful snacks such as nuts, seeds, green shakes, soups, and salads.

4. **Plant-based.** Eat a mostly plant-based diet to reduce inflammation, boost the immune system, prevent diseases, and increase micronutrient and fiber intake. Aim for five

cups of veggies per day or more. The more color on your plate, the better.

5. **Whole foods.** Eat only unprocessed whole food, i.e., vegetables, fruits, nuts, seeds, whole grains, legumes, and unadulterated meats. You'll be eating just like our ancestors did.

6. **Organic.** Buy organic food whenever possible. Visit the Environmental Working Group website http://www.ewg.org for "The Clean 15" and "The Dirty Dozen," lists of produce with the most and least pesticide residue. Also always choose organic corn and soy products to avoid GMOs.

7. **Good Fats.** Consume healthful fats, including olive oil, coconut oil, nuts, seeds, avocado, and omega-3 fatty acids, which can be found in cold-water fish such as wild salmon, and sardines. Healthful fats are essential for vitamin absorption, energy, and a healthy brain and nerves. Avoid inflammatory fats (canola, soy, safflower, and corn oils), which are heavily processed, may cause an unhealthy imbalance of omega-6 to omega-3 fatty acids, and potentially lead to metabolic damage, poor gut health, and inflammation.

8. **Clean proteins.** Choose consciously raised animal proteins such as omega-3 rich organic grass-fed beef, organic pastured chicken and eggs, and wild fish for their lower mercury content. Avoid conventionally farmed

cattle raised in stressful conditions on antibiotics and GMO grain. Plant foods such as beans with rice, quinoa, tofu and tempeh are a good source of protein, too.

9. **Natural.** Avoid processed foods with artificial chemicals, dyes, pesticides, herbicides, added hormones, and antibiotics..

10. **Low sugar.** The recommended amount of added sugar (e.g., in coffee, sweetened drinks, and desserts) for most people is not more than 24 grams or six teaspoons per day, according to the American Heart Association and World Health Organization. Choose fruit and low-glycemic sweeteners such as coconut sugar, maple syrup, and stevia, to avoid sugar spikes. Pass up sugary snacks, desserts, sodas, and even fruit juice. (The sugar may be natural, but it's very concentrated without the fruit fiber).

## A WORD ABOUT SUGAR AND ALCOHOL

Alcohol is quickly broken down into sugar by the body and has the same inflammatory and immune suppressing effects as table sugar, feeding bad gut bacteria and yeast. While alcohol can make us feel relaxed in the moment, it can raise anxiety levels and interfere with sleep, making it difficult to cope with stress in the long run. Eliminating or severely limiting both sugar and alcohol can help you sleep better, improve your mood, reduce harmful gut bacteria, and feel more vital.

As a chocolate lover myself, I know that reducing sugar in your diet can be challenging—especially considering sugar is highly addictive. And depending on how much you've been consuming, you may even experience some withdrawal symptoms, including headaches and cravings. This is normal and is a sign that you are detoxing. Don't worry; the symptoms will soon subside.

11. **Cooking.** Make home-cooked meals, doubling your recipes so you'll have extra to pack for lunch and won't have to dine out. This way you'll know what you're eating; restaurant food is usually not organic and is often cooked with unhealthy oils and excess sodium.

12. **Spice it up.** Add herbs and spices to your cooking to boost your antioxidant intake and aid in detoxing the liver. Plus, herbs and spices make food so much more intensely flavored; you won't miss the junk when your home-cooked food tastes great.

## CLEAN DIET EXERCISE

Your goal is to eat three meals a day, aiming for half a plate of veggies and fruit, a clean protein, and a healthy fat at each meal (see above for food particulars). Here are some guidelines.

1. As you plan your meals, make your shopping lists, stock your shelves, and cook your food, ask yourself: How will this food serve me?

2. Choose a few of your favorite meals. Now, with a little creativity, how will you detoxify them? What ingredients can you swap for healthier ones?

3. Check out the recipes section in Chapter 7 for inspiration and see the gluten and dairy "super substitutes" recipes.

4.  How did you do? Rate each meal for how well you ate clean. Is there anything you can do to clean it up even more next time?

# PART 2. HEALING THROUGH MOOD

You've already given your mood a leg up by detoxing your diet. In part two of the Method, we focus on detoxing the mind by changing thought patterns and using endorphin-boosting exercise to improve how you feel on a daily basis. Much like eating toxic foods, repetitive negative thoughts impact our mood and our overall health. Thanks to the amygdala, a small area of our brains, we are wired to hang on to negative feelings and memories; we remember them better than positive ones. From an evolutionary standpoint, this was an adaptive feature to help us survive, allowing us to remember which predators and poisonous berries to fear and avoid. Our default is to complain, to commiserate, to share what went wrong that day. And misery loves company, right? So negativity spreads and brings everyone down. Because we are hardwired this way, it takes work to shift our attention to what's working and going well. But that's a small price to pay for potentially huge rewards.

Please note that this is not an invitation to blame yourself for your mood or to disregard depression, which may be inherited and can require professional attention. Instead, what you'll find in this section is a wealth of fun exercises that have been proven to make a difference. So much of what we think and feel comes from habit—a set of behaviors, emotional reactions, beliefs, and perceptions that are on autopilot. It takes conscious, intentional action to make changes in our habitual patterns. One example of how to do so is to dispute negative thinking with evidence to the contrary. Think back to times when you were sure that disaster would prevail, only to find that, in fact, nothing bad happened. This weighing of the evidence is especially important for those of us who think in black and white and always/never terms.

It is also important to note that squelching thoughts doesn't work. The mind does not understand *not* thinking about something. For example, when we think, "I am not going to think about having that vanilla latte," that's exactly what we *do* think about. Accordingly, replace, don't erase. Rather than try to ignore certain thoughts, focus on substituting them with new thoughts; think of the healthy smoothie, for instance, versus *not* thinking of the vanilla latte.

This is not all there is to mood and thought rehab. Research shows that gratitude, meditation, love, laughter, and exercise not only increase happiness hormones, but also quell inflammation, and actually turn off genes for certain diseases. Why not try actions with proven positive results in lifting mood? What have you got to lose?

People are drawn to energy. Health, happiness, success, and love each have a certain frequency. That's the energy I believe we are all seeking. So how do we embody it? Our energy, like everything in our lives, is shaped by our perspective. That's good news because that means we can create it. In a lovely little piece of journalism on the website MindBodyGreen.com, the author and meditation expert Jillian Lavender writes about a gardener holding a running hose. When she turns to look and complain about the flourishing weeds, she inadvertently waters them, helping them overtake the garden. Where attention goes, it grows. Where do you put your attention? What energy do you generate?

Similarly, to create the dynamic we want in social interactions, try the practice of "giving what you want." For example, if you want love, give it. If you want good friends, *be* a good friend. When you are dying for a hug, give a hug. We get, and draw to ourselves, what we give.

Put your energy toward the life you seek in order to shift in that direction. After our move to California and near the end of my personal pity party, I began feeling hopeful that I might finally make some new friends. I splurged and joined a nice gym with the intentions of gaining social connections, fitness, and improved mood. When I started going regularly, I met a woman who has been one of the closest friends I've made in my lifetime. Through her, I met a community of women who are like my sisters. To make this change from loneliness to connection, it took changing my focus toward the positive endpoint I sought and away from the loss I suffered. Lesson learned.

Recent research in brain neuroplasticity and the field of positive psychology shows that we can actually increase positive emotions and happiness. Those improvements not only affect how we feel, they affect the impact we have on others. Becoming happier and more positive doesn't mean denying ourselves real emotions of sadness, anger, or frustration. However, we can strengthen the authentic sense of happiness and wellbeing that we were born with. Consider babies. Aren't they naturally confident and happy, free from insecurities, judgments, and the stories we tell ourselves? Somewhere between babyhood and adulthood, our lives become inundated with stress. And mind stress, like food stress, robs us of wellness and our best selves.

Through exercises in positive psychology, we can shift our perspectives to obtain greater peace of mind and joy. With deep breathing and meditation, we can train our brains to notice our ever present mental chatter, the Buddhist so-called "monkey mind" that is on autopilot. By noticing our own thoughts, we can find some distance from them: The space that deep breathing and meditation brings allows us a choice of what to think and feel rather than submit to automatic reactions. My goal in introducing these tools to you is to help you diminish the conflicts in your life and build the kind of positive energy that supports health and wellness.

## STEP 4: PURSUE POSITIVITY

*As you go through the day today, ask yourself this question: What is not wrong? Notice it. Take it in. Allow yourself to be filled.*
- Geneen Roth

According to experts in the field of positive psychology, thriving and flourishing come from resilience, a trait that depends on these key characteristics:
- Goal setting
- Optimism
- Positive role models
- A focus on personal strengths

In addition, research shows that journal writing helps people access their internal emotional world. At the same time it creates physiological changes such as increased blood flow and a boost in immunity. Journal writing can help us access our deepest fears and strengths as well as get clear on our intentions. The following exercises help train the brain to shift toward a positive perspective, one filled with love and gratitude.

**PERSONAL STRENGTHS AND VALUES EXERCISE**

Over the course of a month, using a pen and paper, take a few moments every day to answer one of the questions below. For example, every Monday answer Question 1, every Tuesday answer Question 2, and so on. Repeat this activity each week for four weeks without looking at your answers from the previous week. To get a sense of how your answers may have evolved, compare your daily answers when you are done with the exercise.

1. Monday: What are you good at? Write down as many answers as you can think of.
2. Tuesday: What are your strengths? Write down as many answers as you can think of.
3. Wednesday: Who is your role model? Why? Do you have any similar traits?
4. Thursday: What are your goals for wellness and thriving right now? What did you do within the last week to reach those goals?
5. Friday: Where are you putting your attention? Is your energy focused on the positive goals you seek, or on

negative impediments you believe are preventing you from reaching your objectives?

6.  Saturday: What is most important in your life? How are you honoring that today?

7.  Sunday: How would you like to be remembered? What are you doing today to make sure that comes true?

## GRATITUDE EXERCISES

Research shows that directing our attention to what we are grateful for for 21 days actually rewires the neurons in our brains, enabling us to focus on our blessings and feel happier. Studies also show that gratitude affects us on a hormonal level as well. "By appreciating the colors, aromas, tastes, and textures of food, for instance, we activate important hormones that assist with the digestive process."[23] Further, gratitude increases our production of the neurotransmitters dopamine and serotonin, which is precisely what many prescribed antidepressants do.

There is so much to be grateful for, from the food we get to enjoy to the love we experience. Believe it or not, even pain is something we can be thankful for. Why? Because we are alive to feel it. When I was training for a half marathon last year, my mind was silently screaming, "I can't go on. This hurts. I want to stop!" And then I passed an elderly person in a wheelchair. Boom! Perspective shift. I have legs that can run and lungs that can manage it. How lucky is that?

Here are three easy ways to practice positive thinking and gratitude daily.

1.  **Write down what you're grateful for, which is import-ant for the shift in perspective**. Keep a gratitude journal for 21 days. Every day, either in the morning or at night before bed (or both if you are so inclined), write down several things you are grateful for in your life. As you write, really concentrate on being thankful, how lucky you are, and why. Tune in to your body and find where these positive emotions manifest—your chest, your heart, your shoulders, for example. Feel the gratitude in you. Then, after 21 days, keep going. To bring a fresh daily perspective to gratitude, each morning write down one thing you are looking forward to *that day*. Each night, note at least one thing that happened *that day* that you are grateful for.

2.  **Eat intentionally without distractions.** Notice the food in front of you. Use all of your senses. Chew it slowly. Remember how many billions of people in this world are not as lucky. Be thankful.

3.  **Pay attention to the wonders of your day, the coinci-dences, the delights, the unexpected gifts.** What are you aware of today?

## REFRAMING EXERCISES

When you begin to think negatively, either as a judgment about yourself or someone else—for example, you think you're not good enough or that you're a victim—or you have a fear that something won't work out, try these attitude adjustments:

1. **Notice your negative thinking, then focus on it.** Tune in to your body and become aware of the sensations that arise from your thoughts. Do you feel tight in your chest, acid in your stomach, stress in your shoulders or neck? The more aware you become of your body's signals, the more your body can help you identify that you are in a negative state. This takes practice. Stick with it. The awareness alone helps diminish the power of negative thoughts.

2. **Record in your journal where you tend to manifest negativity and how it feels.** Don't just let the sensations pass by. Write them down so that you can see if there's a pattern.

3. **Look for the good.** Find something positive in that same negative thought sequence. For example, if you are judging other people or yourself, find something you like about them or yourself at the same time. For example, "I'm so forgetful and I'm always late. And I'm very generous and loyal." Turn your attention to the positive thought whenever possible. It sounds Hallmark-y, but it is remarkable how that shift in thought can create a change in your energy and attitude and garner a good response from those around you.

4.   **Focus on the behavior you want to see more of in yourself and in others.** Notice it. Acknowledge it (see the
Acknowledgements Exercise below). Using this positive
approach, one person can single-handedly change a
relationship.

## ACKNOWLEDGMENTS EXERCISE

Place your attention on behaviors you enjoy. Where your energy
goes, it grows. Always coming from the heart, acknowledge
people in your life when they do something positive, thoughtful,
creative, generous, smart, or helpful. Thank them and tell them
you noticed, or that you are grateful. Observe how you feel and
what transpires.

## LOVE MIRROR EXERCISE

This is my mini adaptation of Mirror Work from motivational
author and publisher Louise Hay. To tap into the most loving,
generous part of yourself it's important to feel filled up with love.
You can actually practice loving yourself—here's how: When you
are alone (so you can do this with the utmost conviction) look
at yourself in the mirror. Really look into your own eyes and tell
yourself out loud, "I love you." Do it again and again until you really
hear it and feel moved. How does this feel? Where do you feel it in
your body? Practice this every day for a week. Fill your cup.

**LOVE THY NEIGHBOR EXERCISE**

When you are walking down the street or out for a run, look at someone you are nearing. As you pass them, think of how you essentially came from the same place millions of years ago, the same stardust, the same matter, the same genes. Consider how connected you actually are to this person. We are not islands; we are all already connected. Just by being alive on this planet at the same time, breathing the same air, experiencing the same innovations, news, movies, pop culture, and food we are all connected. Silently, in your own head, think, "I care about you and wish you well." Expect nothing in return from the person you are passing. Watch what happens to the energy between you two. Sometimes, miraculous little connections are made in an instant awash with positive emotions. Repeat this experiment many times, as often as you like, with many different people. What does this do to your own feelings of connection? Does it make you feel as though you're coming from a place of kindness and love?

# STEP 5: WORK EXERCISE INTO YOUR LIFE

*Nothing lifts me out of a bad mood better than*
*a hard workout on my treadmill. It never fails.*
*Exercise is nothing short of a miracle.*
- Cher

There is a good reason fitness is a modern-day "craze." Exercise increases energy, keeps us limber, and helps us sleep. It provides many health benefits as well, including reduced stress, inflammation, cholesterol, blood pressure, and blood sugar; stronger bones and hearts; increased brain cell turnover and blood flow for better memory and productivity; delayed aging; weight loss; and last, but not least, a healthy endorphin release and its accompanying improved mood. It's no wonder, then, that a good workout helps relieve anxiety and depression. Exercise also has the amazing ability to lift us out of a bad day.

My husband and I were once in the middle of a heated argument. As it became clear that we weren't resolving anything and were only building negativity between us, he suggested we go for a run together. When the few miles were up, we were smiling and the argument was long gone. We had completely shifted our energy together.

Research shows that if you make exercise part of your daily regimen (like, eating, sleeping, working) you are more likely to do it. If you are not already exercising, don't beat yourself up about it. A perspective shift about why you would choose to exercise in the first place can help you see working out as a positive activity. For example, shifting your objective from weight loss—which might seem overwhelming or futile—to being healthy is a small change in mindset, but can be very effective. Likewise, shifting from "I *have to* work out" to "I *get to* exercise" puts fitness in a different light.

Keep those long-term objectives in mind, and begin to experiment with different options to find routines you enjoy. Variety is key to keeping it fresh and to finding what feels fun. The best exercise is the one you'll do. In addition, it's important to find your sweet spot. Too much exercise and you can become inflamed and stressed; too little and you don't reap the rewards. For health benefits, exercise at least 30 minutes three times per week. Here are some other tips to help you lead a more active life.

## Find the Exercise You Love

1.  Research shows that we are much more likely to work out in pairs than alone. Find an exercise buddy.
2.  Exercising in nature can help us feel grounded and peaceful. Get outside and walk, hike, bike, swim, or run with a great pair of running shoes. Start small and gradually build. Consider joining a running group and entering some local races (5K to marathon distances) to keep you motivated and give you goals.
3.  Take the stairs instead of elevators. It's a simple action that, when done with regularity, can have fitness benefits.
4.  Try yoga and dance, both great for mind-body awareness and integration. While dance has the benefit of being more socially-oriented, yoga doubles as a moving, breathing meditation, connecting body, mind, and soul. And research shows that yoga reduces chronic pain among many other physiological benefits.[24]
5.  Join a gym and try a variety of options such as spinning, cardio classes, kickboxing and weight training. Find those you enjoy. Maybe you'll also make new friends.

# STEP 6: MEDITATION

*Feelings come and go like clouds in a windy
sky. Conscious breathing is my anchor.*

- Thích Nhất Hạnh

Anytime we focus internally on our breathing or our senses, we have the ability to calm the nervous system and give ourselves some space from our anxious minds. Meditation and mindfulness training, both ancient practices, have been scientifically proven to reduce stress and increase wellbeing. Meditation, a practice of transforming the mind through profound focus, gives us the ability to be less reactive and more intentional in our lives.

Meditation can also help you concentrate better and have a more positive outlook; with meditation you may feel more centered, more calm, and less anxious. It has even been found to alleviate mental health conditions such as depression, attention deficit, and substance abuse. Studies have shown that meditation also has an impact on the amount of gray matter in parts of the brain important for learning, memory, self-awareness, compassion, empathy, and introspection. By enabling us to become the observers of our busy minds and their many thoughts, meditation provides the benefit of mindfulness, or awareness of the mind, and the ability to responsibly choose our behaviors. It allows us to pause and consider whether what we just thought—a judgment, a fear, a concern, an idea—is helpful, misguided, or even worth considering. It helps us see that the ideas in our heads are our own creations. Once we experience this, we have the choice to create a different thought rather than believing the original thought was the absolute truth and the only possibility.

There are many types of meditation, some focusing on breath, some on an internal scan of tension in the body, others on a sound. Some include movement while others do not. The following meditation practices are easy and accessible. Practice them anytime, once or twice daily, in your home, at work, or while traveling (as long as you are not driving!) Most importantly, be kind to yourself, recognizing that there is no one "right" way to meditate. Anytime you take a few minutes to simply breathe quietly, you are practicing self-care and stress reduction.

## SIMPLE DEEP BREATHING

Consciously breathe in through your nose. Exhale more slowly than you inhaled. Practice this throughout your day whenever you are feeling anxious or aware of mounting stress. This simple practice helps me through pressured situations, relieving tension. Deep diaphragmatic breathing (when the belly expands) through the nose signals our sympathetic nervous system (the part involved in the fight or flight response) that we are safe, that there's no saber tooth tiger anywhere in sight, and that we can relax.

## THE 4-7-8 TECHNIQUE

Try a more structured approach to deep breathing by practicing the 4-7-8 technique from Andrew Weil, MD. Sit comfortably in a chair with your eyes closed. Inhale for four seconds, counting silently, "one, two, three, four." Then hold that breath for a count of seven seconds. Next, exhale for a count of eight. Repeat this four times. Notice how you feel. I sometimes use this exercise to help me get to sleep.

## VISUALIZATION

For a meditation with visual imagery, imagine your breath is a wave. As you inhale, picture the water receding from the shore to form the wave. Pause (don't breathe) as the wave crests, then exhale fully (longer than the inhale) as the wave crashes down onto the shore. Begin again.

## MINDFUL MEDITATION

Right now, notice your heart beating in your chest. Are you holding tension in any part of your body? After reading this (or while having someone read it to you slowly as you go), please close your eyes and conduct the following exercise: Sit comfortably with your back supported and feet planted on the floor. Focusing on slow, even breaths through your nose, concentrate on the cool air flowing in and the warm air going out of your nostrils. As thoughts come into your mind, notice them. Without judgment, just watch your thoughts with curiosity, acknowledge them, and let them go. Then return your attention to your breath. Do this for several minutes. Next turn your attention to your body. Continue breathing through your nose. Slowly, beginning with the soles of your feet, conduct a mental scan up your legs, back, belly, neck, arms, shoulders, and head. Notice if you are holding tension as you survey your body, and let it go. Do this for several minutes. End your meditation by focusing on the breath again. Lastly, consider what you are grateful for in regards to your family, your friends, your pets, and yourself. How do you feel?

## TWO-MONTH CHALLENGE

Research shows that it takes an average of 66 days to make a new practice into a habit.[25] Now that you've got the tools you need to improve your wellbeing, continue them for at least two months. Once that time comes to an end, you will likely continue, making them into lifelong habits. A few final thoughts:

1. Stay the course. Continue practicing clean eating and steering clear of food triggers. Incorporate the mood-boosting exercises that you like the best into your daily life.

2. Build momentum. Each of these incremental upgrades to your diet and lifestyle is a form of self-love. Notice how great it feels to take good care of yourself. Self-care is not to be confused with being "selfish." Quite the opposite. The more energy you have, the more you will be able to give of yourself to others, reinforcing the old adage, "You can't pour from an empty cup." Continue adding other self-care practices such as:
   - massages
   - hot baths
   - dry brushing (an Ayurvedic practice for nerve relaxation and lymphatic drainage that involves brushing your dry skin with a long-handled brush in a circular motion from the feet up to your shoulders)
   - lighting soothing candles

- having a quiet cup of tea
- whatever helps you feel loved by you

3. Make time for friends. Connecting with others releases the feel-good hormone oxytocin and helps us feel we are contributing to a community, something larger than ourselves. Research has shown that it requires only 6 to 8 seconds of continuous contact to get our bodies to release oxytocin. Think how much you'll generate with extra long hugs.

4. End conflicts. It's time to close painful conflicts with those you care about by bravely reestablishing communication—but without blaming yourself or the other person and without any expectation of how he or she should react. Use "I" statements such as "I feel sad, isolated, unheard when…", "I miss you when…", and take responsibility by saying "I am sorry." One caveat: This practice should only be undertaken if you feel safe doing so and if it is in your best interest. Re-establishing a toxic relationship or communication is not always healthy or advised.

5. Sleep 7-8 hours. Sleep is the great stabilizer. Get enough to calm your appetite, steady weight-gain hormones, and even out your mood.

## CHAPTER 7

# The Food-Mood Method Shopping Lists and Recipes

Maintaining a diet free from food intolerance triggers and unhealthy additives is a lot easier if you have a properly stocked kitchen and good ideas for home cooking on hand. What follows is a shopping list of healthy staples, a gluten-free guide, and recipes free of the five top food triggers: gluten, dairy, corn, soy, and yeast. They will also help you create dishes free of added sugar. Just one reminder before you begin shopping: Buy organic whenever possible, and choose foods in glass bottles or cans marked "BPA free."

# THE FOOD-MOOD METHOD SHOPPING LIST

**PRODUCE**
Fresh and frozen fruit and veggies, including:

- Artichoke
- Arugula
- Asparagus
- Avocado
- Bok Choy
- Broccoli
- Brussels sprouts
- Cabbage
- Carrots
- Cauliflower
- Celery
- Chicory
- Collard Greens
- Cucumber
- Dandelion Greens
- Endive
- Garlic
- Herbs
- Jicama
- Kale
- Kohlrabi
- Lettuces (Romaine for wraps)
- Mustard Greens
- Mushrooms
- Onion
- Parsnips
- Peas
- Radishes
- Romanesco
- Spinach
- Squashes
- Sweet Potatoes
- Tomatoes
- Zucchini

**REFRIGERATED FOODS**

- Eggs (organic, pastured)
- Fermented veggies (sauerkraut)
- Ghee (clarified butter, considered non-dairy)
- Milks (almond, coconut)

## MEATS

To keep on hand in the freezer:

- Beef (organic, grass-fed)
- Chicken (organic)
- Turkey (ground)

## FROM THE BULK BINS

- Beans
- Grains
- Nuts
- Seeds
- Shredded coconut

## PACKAGED GOODS

- Almond Butter
- Coconut Milk (canned)
- Coconut Oil
- Crackers (gluten- free)*
- Honey (raw)
- Jam (all fruit, no sugar)
- Maple Syrup
- Mayo (organic)
- Mustard
- Oats (gluten-free)
- Olive oil
- Pasta (brown rice)**
- Pesto (olive oil only)
- Seaweed Sheets (nori)***
- Spices
- Tomatoes (canned)****
- Tomato sauce
- Wild salmon (canned)
- Wraps (made of brown rice or dehydrated veggies)

**RECOMMENDED BRANDS**

> \* Crackers: Mary's Gone Crackers; Potter's
>
> \*\* Brown Rice Pasta: Tinkyada; Lundberg
>
> \*\*\* Nori Seaweed: Gimme organic
>
> \*\*\*\* Canned Foods: Muir Glen; Eden; Native Forest

**GLUTEN-FREE GRAINS AND FOODS**

- Almond flour and any nut flour
- Amaranth
- Arrowroot
- Beans, garbanzo bean flour, soy
- Buckwheat
- Corn, cornmeal, cornstarch, polenta
- Garbanzo beans and bean flours
- Millet
- Potatoes, potato flour, potato starch
- Rice, rice flours, rice crackers, risotto
- Sorghum
- Tapioca
- Teff
- Quinoa

## GLUTEN FOODS TO AVOID

Wheat and wheat-containing foods including:

- BBQ sauces
- Bread and bread crumb-containing foods (crab cakes, meatloaf, chicken nuggets, etc.)
- Barley
- Beer
- Bulgur
- Cookies, crackers, cakes
- Couscous
- "Fake" foods such as imitation crab, bacon, and veggie foods
- Farina
- Farro
- Graham, semolina, durum wheats
- Kamut
- Malt flavorings and malt vinegar
- Marinades (some)
- Mustard (beer-containing)
- Oats (except if certified gluten-free)
- Orzo
- Pasta
- Rye
- Soy sauce, and other Asian sauces (teriyaki, oyster, hoisin)
- Spelt
- Tabouli
- Tortillas containing wheat

# Sensitive Recipes

# Thoughtfully designed with food-sensitivities in mind.

🍃 Super Dairy Substitutes
🍃 Fabulous Flour Substitutes
🍃 Balanced Breakfast
🍃 Anti-Inflammatory Appetizers and Snacks
🍃 Soothing Soups, Salads, and Sides
🍃 Excellent Entrees

Most researchers agree that eating a mainly plant-based diet helps boost immunity and prevent diseases. The U.S. Department of Agriculture and Health and Human Services now recommends nine servings of fruits and vegetables daily. This translates to about 2 ½ cups per day for an average adult. The easy way to accomplish this is to fill half your plate with a rainbow of colorful veggies and fruits at each meal, including breakfast! Another way is to add a plant-based protein and super greens supplements to smoothies. The following recipes will also provide you with a wide array of vegetables as well as detoxifying herbs and seaweed.

Gluten, dairy, soy, corn, and yeast are common food triggers and, for that reason, are eliminated from these recipes. Sugar, like other toxins, causes inflammation and makes us more vulnerable to getting illnesses from the common cold to cancer. None of these recipes contains added sugar.

These recipes are designed to help you eat healthfully throughout the day, beginning first thing in the morning. A typical American breakfast of processed, refined carbohydrates, usually in the form of white flour and sugar in bagels, bread, pastry, pancakes, waffles, and sugary cereal, causes blood glucose to spike without the benefit of nutrition. This leaves us quickly depleted, hungry, and moody. In contrast, a breakfast of protein, fiber, and healthful fats will sustain us for hours. Eat well and your body will reward you with long-lasting energy, a clearer mind, a more balanced mood, and even potential weight loss over time.

The protein in these recipes comes from eggs, nuts, seeds, quinoa, vegetables (yes, veggies contain protein), and plant protein powder. Healthful fats come from nuts, seeds, olive oil, coconut oil, avocados, and grass-fed organic ghee or clarified butter used for thousands of years in Ayurvedic medicine to help boost nutrient absorption. Natural fiber-rich fruit is used for sweetness, as is raw honey, maple syrup, or coconut sugar each of which provides the benefit of vitamins and minerals. Super greens are included in smoothie recipes to maximize immune-boosting, detoxifying nutrients. With food sensitivities and health in mind, I've created food trigger-free, nutrient-dense recipes that will keep you balanced and nourished.

# Super Dairy Substitutes

These healthy dairy substitutes for cheese, milk, cream, and sour cream are so delicious, they will likely become your first choice even if dairy isn't your food trigger. Nuts should first be soaked for four hours in water and drained before using in order to remove their coating of phytic acid, and make them easier to digest. When blending the nuts in the recipes, you can play with the amount of water used depending on the consistency of the nut cheeses and creams you prefer.

For butter substitutes in cooking, I use anti-inflammatory fats including olive oil, coconut oil, and avocado oil. Each provides healthy fats, which help our brains and nerves thrive. In some recipes, I use ghee, a nondairy, clarified butter you can find in natural grocery stores.

## ALMOND MILK OR ANY NUT MILK

*You can buy almond milk in stores, but homemade tastes better and is free of gums. If you choose one at your store, make sure it doesn't contain carrageenan, which can cause stomach and intestinal erosion and distress. To make it yourself, you will need a nut milk bag which can be purchased at health food stores and online at Amazon.com.*

**1 c raw almonds (or pecans, cashews, walnuts)**
**4 c water**
**1 t vanilla extract, optional (omit for unflavored almond milk)**

Place all ingredients in a high-powered blender and blend on high speed until very well combined and white. Pour liquid into nut milk bag held over a large bowl or wide-mouth pitcher. Close bag and squeeze slowly until all liquid has been extracted. Keep refrigerated; will last 3-4 days.

## ALMOND "RICOTTA CHEESE"

*With its rich texture, this recipe is a wonderful substitute for traditional ricotta cheese in gluten-free lasagna, tossed with pasta, or as a dessert spooned over fruit with a drizzle of maple syrup.*

**1 c raw almonds**
**1/2 c water**
**1 T fresh lemon juice**
**½ t sea salt**

Place all ingredients in a blender and blend on high speed until creamy. Keep refrigerated; will last 3-4 days.

## HERBED ALMOND CREAM

*This thick, herbal cream is a great substitute for sour cream on baked potatoes, and a dollop is wonderful added to creamy veggie soups such as butternut squash.*

1 c raw almonds
3 T olive oil
1 T fresh lemon juice
1 T fresh chives, chopped
¾ t sea salt
¼ c water

Place all ingredients in a high-powered blender, and blend on high speed until creamy and smooth. Keep refrigerated; will last 3-4 days.

## CASHEW CREAM

*This recipe is so versatile. You can use it in place of cream, melted cheese, or sour cream in both savory and sweet dishes.*

½ c cashew nuts
6 T water
1 T fresh lemon juice
Pinch salt

Place all ingredients in a high-powered blender. Blend on high power until creamy. Scrape nuts down and blend again if needed. Keep refrigerated; will last 3-4 days.

## HORSERADISH ALMOND CREAM

*Spicy, pungent horseradish is a wonderful complement to this sweet nut cream.*

> 1 c raw almonds
> ½ c water
> ¼ c horseradish
> 1 T fresh lemon juice
> 1 T white wine vinegar
> ½ t sea salt

Place all ingredients in a high-powered blender and blend on high speed until creamy and smooth. Keep refrigerated; will last 3-4 days.

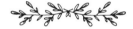

## KALE PESTO

*This is a delicious way to eat kale. It is so good it doesn't need the Parmesan cheese found in classic pesto.*

> ½ head Lacinato kale leaves, stems removed
> ½ c sunflower seeds, toasted
> ½ c fresh basil leaves
> ¼ c olive oil
> ½ t salt
> 1 clove garlic

Place all ingredients in a blender and blend on high speed until creamy and smooth. Keep refrigerated; will last 3-4 days.

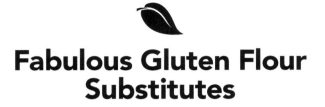

# Fabulous Gluten Flour Substitutes

### GLUTEN FREE FLOUR

*I buy these flours from the bulk section of my health food store and combine them in a big airtight container when I get home. That way I have a quantity of gluten-free flour whenever I need it and save money making it myself.*

> 2 c brown rice flour
> 1 c white rice flour
> 1 c quinoa flour
> 1 c tapioca flour

Pour all flours into container.  Mix very well with a large spoon, or close container tightly and shake well. Store in a cool place.

### GLUTEN FREE "BREAD" CRUMBS

*These crumbs can be used in any savory recipe calling for bread crumbs. I use them mixed in with meat loaf and as a coating for chicken nuggets.*

> 2 c organic brown rice crisps (check labels for lowest sugar content)
> ¼ c chia seeds

1 T dried onion flakes
1 T dried thyme
1 T dried oregano
2 t garlic powder
1 t salt
½ t dried red pepper flakes
½ t freshly ground pepper

Combine all ingredients in a bowl. Transfer to an airtight container and store in the refrigerator.

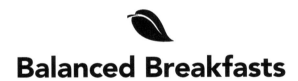

# Balanced Breakfasts

### VEGGIE FRITTATA

*My good friend Dorothea is Italian. Her family is from Sestri Levante, a town in Liguria where they make these beautiful, thin delicacies. She taught me how to make frittatas this way.*

*Serves 2*

> **3 T olive oil, divided**
> **¼ yellow onion, chopped**
> **2 c fresh spinach leaves or 1 ½ cups zucchini, chopped into small cubes**
> **2 T fresh basil or cilantro, chopped**
> **2 eggs**
> **Pinch salt and freshly ground pepper**

Warm 1 tablespoon of the olive oil over medium heat in an 11" sauté pan, Add the onion and sauté until it begins to turn golden brown, about 5 minutes. Add onion and spinach or zucchini. Continue cooking, stirring, until wilted. If using zucchini, cook until soft, about 5 minutes. Turn off heat. Add herbs and stir.

In a small bowl, beat eggs. Add salt and pepper and stir. Stir the cooked veggies into the bowl of eggs and mix well until combined. Pour the remaining 2 tablespoons of the olive oil into the sauté pan and warm over medium-low heat, spreading to coat pan. Add egg mixture to pan and spread out thinly. Cook until edges become golden brown, about 5 minutes.

Using a round plate, cover frittata in pan. Carefully turn pan over to release the eggs onto the plate. The browned side should now be face up on plate. Slide frittata back into pan, uncooked side down. Continue cooking another 5 minutes. Serve immediately or at room temperature.

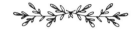

## BANANA-ALMOND PANCAKES

*These pancakes are a delicious breakfast or afternoon snack. I'll often make a double batch and keep leftovers in the fridge for later. Cooked in coconut oil, the edges become crisp and the flavor has a hint of coconut. Substitute grass-fed organic ghee or butter if you are not a coconut fan. The chia seeds in this recipe are loaded with soluble fiber, and are great for digestion and lowering cholesterol.*

*Makes 8 small pancakes*

> 1 heaping T coconut oil
> 2 ripe bananas
> 1 heaping T almond butter
> 1 egg, beaten
> 1 t ground cinnamon
> 1 T chia seeds
> Berries, optional

Melt the coconut oil in a large sauté pan over medium heat. Meanwhile, mash the bananas in a bowl. Add the almond butter and combine. Stir in the egg. Add the cinnamon and chia seeds and mix well. Drop generous tablespoons of batter into the pan. Keep heat medium to medium-low as these will burn if cooked too quickly. After 4-5 minutes, or when edges begin to brown, flip pancakes and cook on the other side. If desired, serve topped with berries.

## CINNAMON GRANOLA

*Most store-bought granola is made with canola or other unhealthy oils. By making it yourself, you choose the ingredients. This one is made with health-boosting coconut oil and gluten-free oats among other goodies.*

*Fills two large Mason, Ball, or Atlas jars*

> 2 T coconut oil
> 2 c gluten-free oats (I use Bob's Red Mill brand)
> 1 T ground cinnamon
> 1 c sunflower seeds
> 1 c unsalted almonds
> 1 c unsweetened shredded coconut
> ¾ c dried cherries
> 2 T maple syrup

Preheat oven to 350°. Place coconut oil, oats, and cinnamon on cookie sheet. Use your hands or spatula and combine well. Bake for 10-15 minutes, stirring occasionally, until light golden brown. Add sunflower seeds and almonds to the mix. Combine well and spread the granola out so it's in a single layer. Continue baking for 5 minutes. Add coconut in single layer on top. Bake 3-5 minutes more, watching carefully as the coconut shreds brown quickly. Remove pan from oven. Add cherries and syrup. Stir well, then let cool before serving.

## CREAMY ALMOND KALE SMOOTHIE

*This smoothie is loaded with nutrient goodness. Kale is high in vitamins and minerals; bananas are high in fiber and minerals; and almond butter adds protein and healthy fat. Delicious any time of day. Cheers!*

*Serves 2*

> 1 c almond milk (store-bought organic or homemade, see page 139)
> 1 c kale leaves pulled from stems (or substitute spinach leaves or favorite greens)
> 1 banana
> 1 heaping T almond butter
> 1 scoop unflavored or Yerba Mate flavored RAW protein powder, or other organic plant protein, optional

Place all ingredients in a blender and blend until smooth.

## TROPICAL CHOCOLATE SMOOTHIE

*This smoothie is rich and creamy like a chocolate ice cream shake and can be served for breakfast or as a healthy dessert. One of its prime ingredients, coconut oil helps balance hormones, provides healthful fat for optimal brain and nerve function, and is also anti-bacterial. The organic powders provide plant protein, fiber, essential vitamins, minerals, and health-promoting phytonutrients.*

*Serves 1*

½ c almond milk (store-bought organic or homemade; see page 139)
½ c frozen strawberries
1 banana
1 heaping T almond butter
1 T coconut oil
1 scoop chocolate RAW plant-based protein powder
1 scoop chocolate Greens Superfood plant-based nutrition powder

Place all ingredients in a blender and blend until smooth.

## SAUERKRAUT EGG

*Take your simple egg and do it one better. Fermented sauerkraut replaces salt, adding tangy, briny flavor and gut-healthy probiotics.*

*Serves 1*

1 T olive oil
1 cup packed spinach leaves
1 egg
1 T sauerkraut

Warm the olive oil in a large sauté pan over medium heat. Add the spinach and sauté for a few minutes, stirring occasionally, until wilted. Remove spinach and place on a plate. Without cleaning the pan, crack the egg into the pan and cook until whites are solid enough to flip, a minute or two. Flip the egg and cook for 10 seconds. Turn off heat. Let egg continue to cook for about 30 seconds. Remove egg, place on top of spinach and top with sauerkraut. Serve immediately.

## OAT-MEGA

*This oatmeal packs a lot of omega-3 fatty acids, minerals, and fiber into one bowl. Both chia seeds and walnuts are omega-3 stars and Brazil nuts provide thyroid-healthy selenium. If desired, serve topped with fresh berries and other fruit.*

*Serves 1*

> 1 c almond milk (store-bought organic or homemade nut milk)
> ½ c gluten-free oats (I use Bob's Red Mill)
> ¼ c walnuts
> 4 Brazil nuts
> 1 generous T chia seeds
> 1 generous T unsweetened shredded coconut, toasted
> 1 t maple syrup, optional

In a small saucepan, combine almond milk and oats. Heat to boiling over high heat, then lower to medium. Continue cooking until desired consistency, from 5-15 minutes. Pour into bowl. Sprinkle with remaining ingredients and serve.

## AMAZING HEALTH BREAD

*Adapted from Food52.com*

*This bread is so easy and fun to make. You can be creative, trying different nuts and dried fruits, adding puréed or diced fresh fruits, and tinkering with different grains and flours. Psyllium husk is high in soluble fiber, and great for digestion and lowering cholesterol. You can find organic psyllium husk in health food markets. Avoid non-organic as it is loaded with pesticide.*

*Makes 1 loaf*

> 2 c shelled sunflower seeds
> 1 c flaxseed meal
> 1 c almonds or walnuts
> 1 ½ c gluten-free rolled oats (I use Bob's Red Mill)
> 1 ½ c almond meal
> 1 c shredded coconut
> 1 c dried currants or cranberries
> ¼ c chia seeds
> ½ c psyllium seed husks (6 T if using psyllium husk powder)
> ½ t sea salt
> 6 T melted coconut oil or ghee or combination
> 3 c water

In a large mixing bowl, combine all dry ingredients, stirring well. Whisk maple syrup, oil, and water together in a measuring cup. Add to the dry ingredients and mix very well until everything is completely soaked and dough becomes very thick. Pour mixture into a flexible, silicon loaf pan or a standard loaf pan lined with parchment. Smooth the top of loaf with the back of a spoon. Let sit on the counter for at least 2 hours.

After 2 hours, preheat oven to 350°. Place loaf pan in the oven on the middle rack, and bake for 30 minutes. Remove bread from loaf pan, place it upside down directly on the rack, carefully peeling away parchment paper, and bake for another 30 to 40 minutes. Bread is done when it sounds hollow when tapped. Let cool completely before slicing. Best when sliced thinly and toasted for extra crispiness. Store bread in a tightly sealed container in refrigerator for up to five days or in freezer.

## PUMPKIN BUCKWHEAT PORRIDGE

*Though its name may be misleading, buckwheat is a gluten-free, highly nutritious grain. It is loaded with magnesium and rich in iron, fiber and other minerals.*

*Serves 2*

> 1 c buckwheat or "kasha" or gluten-free rolled oats
> 1 ¼ c almond milk (store-bought organic or homemade nut milk, see page 139) or coconut milk, divided
> ½ cup pumpkin puree (I use canned organic)
> 1 t cinnamon
> ½ t ginger
> ⅛ t cloves
> ⅛ t sea salt
> 2 T ground chia seeds
> 2-3 T raw honey or maple syrup
> ¼ c walnuts, chopped
> 2 T shredded coconut, toasted

If you bought kasha, you've got pre-toasted buckwheat grains. If you bought buckwheat, toast one cup in a sauté pan over medium heat for 5 minutes, stirring often, to bring out the nutty flavor of the grains.

In a saucepan, combine 1 cup water, 1 cup of the almond milk, and buckwheat or oatmeal. Bring to a boil, then stir in the pumpkin puree, cinnamon, ginger, cloves, and salt. Turn down the heat to a simmer and cook for 15-20 minutes. Once the liquid has evaporated, turn off heat and stir in chia seeds.

To serve, divide the porridge between two bowls and add remaining ¼ cup almond milk or more or less if desired. Top with honey or maple syrup, walnuts, and coconut.

## PROTEIN RICE PUDDING

*This multigrain pudding is high in protein and fiber. It is a healthier version of classic rice pudding and is lightly sweetened with figs and maple syrup.*

*Serves 4-5 for breakfast or dessert*

> **1 T ghee or butter**
> **1 T olive oil**
> **1 c Arborio rice**
> **3 c almond milk, warmed (store-bought organic or homemade nut milk)**
> **¼ c red quinoa**
> **12 dried figs, covered and soaked in boiling filtered water for ½ hour**
> **½ t cardamom**
> **3 T pure maple syrup**
> **2 t chia seeds**
> **¼ c Cashew Cream (see page 140)**

In a medium saucepan, melt ghee. Add olive oil. Add Arborio rice and stir to coat. Cook for a minute until rice edges become translucent. Add ½ cup of the almond milk to the rice and stir often until absorbed. Add another ½ cup and repeat. Continue process until all almond milk has been added and absorbed. Turn off heat.

Cook quinoa: In a small saucepan, combine quinoa and ½ c water. Gently boil for 12 minutes. Add cooked quinoa to rice. Puree figs with in a high-powered blender. Add fig puree, cardamom, maple syrup, chia seeds, and Cashew Cream to rice-quinoa mixture. Stir until well combined. Cool in refrigerator. Eat cooled or at room temperature.

## SEAWEED BREAKFAST WRAP

*Seaweed is an excellent source of iodine, which is vitally important for thyroid function. Combined with avocado, eggs, and umeboshi plum paste, this wrap provides many essential nutrients for brain health and disease prevention. Note: Fermented umeboshi plums are rich in antioxidants, probiotics, and used as a digestive aid in Japan.*

*Serves 1*

> Olive oil or coconut oil
> 2 eggs
> 1 sheet nori seaweed (my favorite brand is Gimme organic seaweed as it is crispy and oversized)
> ½ t umeboshi plum paste
> ½ ripe avocado, sliced thin
> 1 small handful fresh baby spinach leaves
> 1 T fresh cilantro, chopped (or other herb)

Briefly heat oil in a medium pan over medium heat. Crack and scramble eggs in bowl and add to pan, stirring until cooked through.

Lay seaweed sheet on a plate. Spread a ½-inch line of plum paste down the left edge of the seaweed, facing up. In the center of the sheet, evenly place scrambled egg, and top with avocado, spinach, and cilantro, leaving room on both sides to wrap the sheet over the egg mixture. Fold right side of sheet over egg mixture. Fold left side over and press plum paste edge to seal the wrap. Slice in half, and eat while warm.

# Anti-Inflammatory Appetizers and Snacks

### GUACAMOLE

*This simple version of guacamole makes a great appetizer for guests or anytime snack. Serve with raw sliced jicama, radishes, cucumbers, and other crunchy veggies.*

**3 ripe avocados**
**Juice of 1 large lemon**
**¼ t salt (I prefer Himalayan), or to taste**

Scoop avocado into bowl. Add lemon juice and salt. Use potato masher or hands to combine until smooth. Serve immediately.

### HUMMUS

*This creamy, protein- and fiber-rich hummus was my mother's classic recipe. Serve with raw sliced carrots, cucumber, radishes and/or jicama.*

**1 20-ounce can of chickpeas (or 2 15-oz cans), drained and well rinsed**
**¼ cup lemon juice**
**½ cup olive oil**
**1 clove garlic**
**½ t freshly ground black pepper**
**Salt to taste**

Place all ingredients in food processor and blend until creamy. Store in an airtight container in the refrigerator.

## KALE CHIPS

*Rich in protein, fiber, and vitamins, kale has become trendy—one of the better trends, if you ask me. These chips enticed my kids to love the healthful vegetable.*

**1 head Dino or Lacinato kale**
**Olive oil**
**¼ t salt**

Preheat oven to 350°. Wash and dry the kale leaves until they are very dry. Holding one kale stem at a time, pull leaves away from stem in one unzipping motion. Discard stems. Rub the leaves with oil so that they are completely covered back and front, and place on sheet pan. Using your fingers, sprinkle leaves with salt.

Bake for 10-15 minutes, watching to be sure they do not burn.

## CRAB CEVICHE

*Clean and fresh, this ceviche requires a little advanced planning as well as some prep work. The results are well worth the effort, and it makes an impressive dish for a party.*

*Serves 8*

1 lb fresh crabmeat
Zest and juice of 2 oranges
Zest and juice of 2 lemons
Zest and juice of 2 limes
½ c olive oil
½ red onion, finely chopped
1 jalapeno pepper, seeded and finely chopped
⅓ c cilantro leaves, finely chopped
Salt and freshly ground pepper to taste
1 c orange or tangerine segments, chopped

In a large non-reactive ceramic or glass bowl, combine zest, juices, olive oil, onion, jalapeno, cilantro, salt and pepper. Stir well and add crabmeat. Stir again until marinade completely covers crab. Cover bowl and place in refrigerator for 2 hours. Drain crab mixture in a colander discarding liquid. Add orange segments, stir, and serve.

## SPINACH DIP

*Delightful with raw veggies, this dip requires some advanced preparation to allow it to chill in the refrigerator.*

10 oz package frozen spinach, thawed
1 c Cashew Cream (see page 140)
½ c green onion, chopped
½ c fresh parsley, chopped
½ t fresh dill, chopped
½ t dried oregano
Juice of ½ lemon
½ t seasoned salt

In a medium bowl, blend all ingredients with a spoon. Refrigerate for 3 hours before serving.

## FARINATA – GARBANZO BEAN CRISP

*This easy Italian snack, a crispy chickpea pancake, is delicious served alone or with a dip such as the Horseradish Almond Cream (see page 141) or with the cold cucumber soup.*

- 1 c garbanzo bean flour
- 1 c water
- 4 T olive oil
- 2 t dried thyme leaves
- 1 t salt
- 1 shallot, chopped finely

Preheat oven to 450°. Once heated, place a 12" ovenproof skillet in the center of the oven for about 5 minutes, or until very hot. Meanwhile combine garbanzo bean flour, water, 2 tablespoons olive oil, thyme, salt, and shallot in medium bowl and whisk well. Pull hot pan out of oven. Pour remaining 2 tablespoons of olive oil into pan and swirl until pan is fully coated. Pour batter into pan and swirl until evenly distributed. Bake in the center of the oven for 15-20 minutes, or until edges are golden brown.

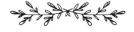

## NAN'S BANANA WALNUT DOMES

*These domes are a great substitute for bars on the go. They are loaded with powerful nutrients. One or two of them also makes a healthy, satisfying dessert.*

*Makes about 40 cookies*

18 dates, pitted
1 large banana
½ c gluten-free quick-cooking oats
½ c almond meal
½ c shredded coconut
¼ c coconut sugar
¼ c flaxseed meal
2 t ground cinnamon
½ t salt
½ t baking powder
½ c walnut pieces

Preheat oven to 325° convection setting preferred. Line a cookie sheet with parchment paper.

In a food processor, place the dates and process until combined into a paste. They will form a ball as they process. Remove from processor and set aside. Puree the banana in the processor until smooth. In the bowl of a large mixer, combine the remaining ingredients and mix on low speed until well combined. Add dates and banana to the bowl and mix on low-medium speed until well incorporated.

Using a small ice cream scoop (#70), scoop batter and place domes on the lined cookie sheet, making six rows of five. If you don't have a scoop, use rounded tablespoons of batter and form into balls with your hands before placing on the cookie sheet. (They will not spread during baking.) Bake 13 minutes. Best eaten warm or at room temperature. Store in an airtight container in the refrigerator.

## NAN'S SWEET POTATO CHOCOLATE CHIP DOMES

*These domes won first place in Tyler Florence's Sprout baby food contest using his pureed sweet potato. They are a great substitute for bars on the go and make a yummy dessert.*

*Makes 47 cookies*

> **18 dates, pitted**
> **½ c gluten-free quick-cooking oats**
> **½ c almond meal**
> **¼ c coconut sugar**
> **¼ c flaxseed meal**
> **2 T ground cinnamon**
> **½ t dried powdered ginger**
> **½ t baking powder**
> **½ t salt**
> **¼ t ground cloves**
> **½ c dried currants**
> **½ c sweet potato puree \***
> **1 t vanilla extract**
> **¾ c dark chocolate chips (70% chocolate)**

Preheat oven to 300°, convection setting preferred. Line a cookie sheet with parchment paper. In a food processor, place the dates and process until combined into a paste. They will form a ball as they process. In the bowl of a large mixer, combine the next nine ingredients and mix on low speed until well combined. Add the dates to the bowl and mix on low-medium speed until well incorporated. Stir in the currants until they're coated, separated, and integrated into the batter. Add the sweet potato and vanilla, and mix on low-medium speed until just incorporated. Stir in chocolate chips until evenly incorporated.

Using a small ice cream scoop (#70), scoop batter and place domes on the lined cookie sheet, making six rows of five. If you don't have a scoop, use rounded tablespoons of batter and form into balls with hands before placing on the cookie sheet. (They will not spread during baking.) Bake 18 minutes. Best eaten warm or at room temperature. Store in a sealed container in the refrigerator.

*Note: You can buy organic canned sweet potato puree, or bake a sweet potato. To bake, poke holes in sweet potato with fork and bake at 350° on sheet pan for an hour or until soft; scoop out ½ cup of sweet potato.

## COCONUT CACAO CHIA PUDDING

*Between the dates and the chia seeds, this pudding is loaded with fiber. Chia is also high in calcium, magnesium, and heart-healthy omega-3 fatty acids. Great as is, or serve with sliced strawberries.*

*Serves 3*

> 1 can full fat coconut milk
> 3 T cocoa powder
> 2 T raw honey
> 3 fresh dates, pitted
> 1 t ground cinnamon
> ½ t vanilla
> 3 T chia seeds
> 2 t cacoa nibs

Place first six ingredients in a blender. Blend on high speed for 20-30 seconds until well combined and dates are pulverized. Add the chia seeds and cacao nibs and stir with a spatula to combine. Pour mixture into three small containers such as jam jars or mini bowls. Refrigerate for 30 minutes or more before serving.

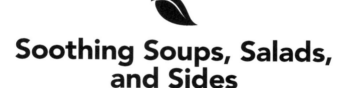

# Soothing Soups, Salads, and Sides

## BUTTERNUT SQUASH SOUP

*Butternut squash is loaded with vitamin A, many of the B vitamins, and fiber. The flexibility of this recipe allows you to choose how rich and creamy you would like the soup to be.*

*Serves 8*

> 6 c chicken broth
> 1 c onion, thinly sliced
> 1 clove garlic, minced
> ½ t thyme
> ¼ t pepper
> 2 ½ c butternut squash, peeled, seeded, and cubed
> 1 c almond milk (see page 139); for a richer soup, use canned coconut milk)
> ¼ to ½ t salt
> ½ c parsley, finely chopped
> Herbed Almond Cream (see page 140), optional

Bring broth to a boil in a large pot. Add onion, garlic, thyme, pepper, and butternut squash cubes; bring to a second boil. Reduce heat and simmer, uncovered, for 40 minutes. Transfer soup to a blender or food processor and puree; return to pot. Reduce heat to simmer and add almond milk. Taste and adjust seasonings. Simmer 10 more minutes. To serve, garnish with parsley and, if desired, a dollop of Herbed Almond Cream.

## QUINOA "MATZO" BALL SOUP

*There are many variations on chicken soup recipes handed down in Jewish families. This one, from my mother-in-law, is my all-time favorite. The longer it simmers, the richer the flavor. I make it on a Sunday afternoon or on a day when I'm working at home and have time to let it simmer for 3 hours.*

Serves 8

> 3 organic chicken breasts on the bone, skin removed
> 1 onion, ends cut off, skin on, cut in half
> 3 large parsnips, cleaned, trimmed and cut into large chunks
> 1 bunch celery, cleaned, trimmed and cut into large chunks
> 4 large carrots, cleaned, trimmed and cut into large chunks
> 1 bunch parsley
> 1 t salt
> ½ t freshly ground pepper
> 6 cups organic chicken broth or water
> Gluten-Free Quinoa "Matzo" Balls (see following recipe)

Place all ingredients except "matzoh" balls in a large soup or pasta pot. Place lid on the pot and bring soup to boil over med-high heat. Turn heat down to low and simmer for 3 hours.

Place a colander over a large bowl and strain soup. Return soup to the pot. Return carrots to pot, cutting them into smaller pieces if desired. Pull chicken off the bone, shred, and return to pot if desired. Otherwise, save chicken for chicken salad or chicken tostadas (See

Excellent Entrees section for recipes). Add "matzoh" balls to the soup and serve.

## GLUTEN-FREE QUINOA "MATZO" BALLS

*Note: These are not intended for Passover as they contain baking powder, a leavening agent.*

- 1 c quinoa flakes
- ½ t aluminum free baking powder
- ½ t xanthan gum
- 1 t salt
- ½ t freshly ground pepper
- ¼ c olive oil
- 3 eggs, separated
- 1 t fresh parsley, chopped

In a large mixing bowl, combine the first five ingredients. Mix well. In a small bowl, whisk together the olive oil, egg yolks and parsley. Pour the wet ingredients into the dry ingredients and combine until all the quinoa flakes are moistened. In a medium to large size mixing bowl, beat the egg whites until just stiff; do not beat to the dry peak stage as you would for meringues. Fold the egg whites into the batter and gently combine until all the quinoa is moist, loose, and without clumps. Let sit for 20 minutes in the refrigerator.

Meanwhile bring a large pot of water to a boil. Reduce heat to a gentle boil. Using a teaspoon, scoop up rounded spoonfuls of the batter and shape into small balls with your hands. Gently drop the balls into the gently boiling water. When all balls have been added to the water, flip each ball over with a spoon and cook covered for 20 minutes. Use a slotted spoon to lift and drain the balls before adding to the chicken soup.

## ZUCCHINI BASIL SOUP

*This easy soup is special enough to serve at a party. High in vitamin C, manganese, and fiber, zucchini is a healthful, delicious, and versatile squash. Basil and wine impart hints of their unique flavors. If you find you can tolerate dairy, Parmesan cheese can be substituted for the Cashew Cream.*

*Serves 4-6*

>     2 T olive oil
>     ¾ c onion, chopped
>     2 garlic cloves, chopped
>     2 lbs zucchini, trimmed and cut into 2" pieces
>     1 t salt
>     4 c chicken broth*
>     1 c white wine
>     ½ c basil leaves, packed
>     ¼ c Cashew Cream (see page 140)
>     Salt
>     Freshly ground pepper

Place oil in a 4-quart pot or saucepan. Add onion and garlic and cook over medium heat for about 5 minutes or until translucent. Add zucchini and salt and cook 5 minutes more, stirring occasionally. Add broth and wine. Cover and simmer until tender, about 15 minutes. Turn off heat. Add basil to wilt, and blend with an immersion blender or in two batches in a regular blender. Season with salt and pepper to taste.

To serve, pour soup into bowls, and top with dollop of Cashew Cream.

*Note: For homemade chicken broth, see chicken soup recipe in first half of Quinoa "Matzo" Ball Soup (see page 164). Otherwise, use organic packaged broth.

## MISO LENTIL SOUP

*This hearty soup requires some advanced preparation to soak the lentils. The lentils and brown rice in this soup provide complete proteins. Add a salad, and you've got a meal. Fermented and organic soy, such as that in miso, is the healthiest way to eat soybeans. Organic is best—it means it's not GMO soy.*

Serves 6-8

> 1 T olive oil
> 1 yellow onion, diced
> 4 carrots, diced
> 1 c pink lentils, dried
> 2 T brown rice miso
> ¼ c brown rice
> 6 c vegetable broth (or chicken broth)

Cover lentils with cold water and soak for four hours or more. They will double in size. When done, drain lentils. In a medium stockpot, heat the olive oil, onions, and carrots over medium heat. Cook until onions are soft. Add the lentils, rice, miso, and broth. Stir well to combine. Bring to a boil, then reduce heat to a simmer. Cover, and cook for 30 minutes, stirring occasionally. Serve hot.

## MUSHROOM SOUP

*I adapted this recipe from Ina Garten's delicious and rich mushroom soup. Here, even without cream, this soup is hearty and delicious. By puréeing the mushroom stems and carrots in the mushroom stock, the result is a deeply flavored, creamy soup base with delicious bites of mushroom caps. If you prefer a smooth soup, you can puree the entire pot.*

*Serves 4-6*

>    5 ounces fresh shiitake mushrooms
>    5 ounces fresh cremini mushrooms
>    5 ounces fresh white mushrooms
>    2 T olive oil, divided
>    2 T ghee, divided
>    1 cup leeks, well washed and chopped
>    1 carrot, chopped
>    ½ c yellow onion, chopped
>    5 sprigs fresh thyme plus 2 t thyme leaves
>    2 t salt, divided
>    1 ½ pepper, divided
>    6 c organic vegetable stock
>    ¼ c gluten free flour (see page 142)
>    1 c dry white wine
>    ½ c minced fresh flat-leaf parsley

Rinse and gently tumble all mushrooms in a colander. (It is a myth that they soak up water.) Shake off water. Separate the stems from the caps. Coarsely chop stems. Slice the mushroom caps into ¼ inch thick slices. If they are very wide, cut them into bite-sized pieces. Set aside.

In a large stockpot, heat 1 T of the olive oil and 1 T of the ghee. Add the chopped mushroom stems, the leeks, carrot, sprigs of thyme, 1 t salt, and ½ t pepper, and cook over medium-low heat for 10 to 15 minutes, or until the vegetables are soft. Add the stock, bring to a boil, then reduce the heat and simmer uncovered for 30 minutes. Turn off the heat. Remove thyme stems, and carefully purée the hot soup using an immersion blender or, in batches, a regular blender. You should have about 5 cups of stock.

In a large sauté pan, heat the remaining 1 T olive oil and 1 T ghee and add the onion. Cook over low heat for 15 to 20 minutes, or until the onion begins to brown. Add the sliced mushroom caps and cook for another 10 minutes, or until the caps are browned and tender. Add in the flour, stir to combine, and cook for 1 minute. Add the white wine and stir for another minute, scraping the bottom of the pot. Next, add the mushroom mixture to the mushroom stock. Add 1 t salt, and 1 t pepper and stir well. Reduce the heat and simmer for 5 minutes. To serve, garnish with the parsley.

## THAI MEATBALL SOUP

*I created this soup one night when I was feeling a cold coming on. The Thai lime and coconut combination has always felt soothing. Plus, it's an easy, healthful meal in a bowl.*

*Serves 4*

For the meatballs:
- 1 lb ground dark meat turkey or chicken
- 1 T dried onion flakes
- 1 t dried thyme
- 1 t dried oregano
- 1 t curry powder
- 3 T ground flax meal
- 1 t salt
- ½ t pepper

For the soup:
- 2 T olive oil
- 1 large onion, chopped
- 3 stalks celery, chopped
- ¼ c white wine, optional
- 1 16 oz box organic vegetable broth
- 3 patty pan squash, cut into 1 inch cubes
- 1 parsnip, cut into 1 inch pieces
- 1 can organic coconut milk
- Juice of 2 limes
- ½ t salt
- 1 c baby spinach leaves
- 1 large leaf Swiss chard, chopped, including stem
- ½ package brown rice pasta
- 1 avocado, peeled, seeded and cubed into ½" pieces
- 1 T cilantro, chopped

To make the meatballs, combine all the ingredients in a large bowl and mix well. Using your hands, form into 1-inch round balls. Set aside.

In a large soup pot, heat olive oil over medium heat. Add onion and celery and cook, stirring occasionally, until onions are translucent and beginning to brown. Add meatballs, nestling them between the veggies so they touch the bottom of the pot. Cook meat, turning balls with a spoon until they are seared on all sides. Add the wine, stir, and cook for a few minutes. Add the vegetable broth, squash, and parsnip to pot and stir. Cover pot, bring to boil, and reduce heat to simmer for 20 minutes.

Add the coconut milk, lime juice, and salt to the broth. Stir well to combine and continue cooking for 10 minutes more or until heated through. When finished, turn off heat.

Meanwhile, in separate pot, bring water to a boil, and cook brown rice pasta according to package directions. Drain pasta and add to broth along with the spinach and Swiss chard; stir well. To serve, ladle into bowls. Top with avocado and cilantro.

## COLD CUCUMBER SOUP

*This is my tweaked version of a cream-based recipe. I have replaced dairy with coconut milk and included Cashew Cream for a rich, delicious cold soup. If you find you can tolerate dairy, sheep's milk yogurt is a tangy addition in place of the Cashew Cream.*

1 c Cashew Cream (see page 140)
1.5 c coconut milk
2 cucumbers, peeled and chopped
½ c fresh mint leaves
¼ c fresh dill
½ c lemon juice
½ t salt

Place all ingredients, adding salt to taste, into a food processor. Pulse a few times until cucumbers are chopped but not mushy. Chill in the refrigerator until ready to serve.

## KALE SALAD WITH MISO TAHINI

*Adapted from NavitasNaturals.com*

*The pungent flavors and creaminess of this dressing are great accompaniments to the slightly bitter, chewy kale. Tahini, a paste made from sesame seeds and high in healthful fats, calcium, and B vitamins, and kale, high in protein, fiber, many nutrients, vitamins, and minerals, is a powerhouse combination.*

*Serves 1 as an entrée*

1 T tahini
1 T miso paste
1 T lemon juice
1 garlic clove, minced
1 t ginger, minced
1-2 T water
3 c bite-sized organic kale pieces from about
10 medium-sized leaves, stemmed and torn

To make dressing, combine tahini, miso, lemon juice, garlic and ginger in a small bowl or measuring cup; mix well. Add water until consistency is creamy. Place kale in a salad bowl and toss with the dressing. Using your hands, massage the dressing into kale leaves for a minute to soften leaves.

## CRUNCHY ASIAN BUCKWHEAT SALAD

*This might be my favorite salad of all time, and the ingredients are stunningly healthy. For instance, despite its name, buckwheat is unrelated to wheat and is a gluten-free, high-fiber grain. This salad is also made with crunchy and satisfying romaine, a nutrient-dense lettuce, high on the ANDI scale (see Chapter 5). Another ingredient, seaweed, provides much needed iodine, and the anchovies are rich in omega-3 fatty acids. (I use imported anchovy paste in a tube, which will keep in the fridge for several weeks.) And there's more: Tahini, made from sesame seeds, contains healthful fat and is high in calcium. When buying miso, opt for organic to avoid GMO soy.*

*Serves 2-3 as an entrée*

> 1 head Romaine lettuce
> 3 T nori seaweed, finely sliced
> Juice of 1 lemon
> 1 t red wine vinegar
> 1 t rice vinegar
> 1 t tamari or gluten free soy sauce
> 2 T organic brown miso paste
> 3 T tahini paste
> 1-2 t anchovy paste

3 T olive oil
½ c kasha or whole buckwheat grain
3 T sesame seeds, toasted

Slice lettuce into bite size pieces. Place in a salad bowl and add the seaweed. In a separate bowl, combine the next seven ingredients and mix well. Divide mixture in half. Keep one half in the bowl and store the other half in fridge for another salad.

In a medium sauté pan, heat the olive oil over medium heat. Add the buckwheat and sesame seeds and sauté for about 5 minutes, or until the grains becomes golden brown. Pour hot mixture and its oil into the dressing in the bowl. Stir while sizzling. Scoop dressing onto salad and toss well. Serve immediately.

## BAKED SWEET POTATO FRIES

*This healthier baked version of French fries is made with sweet potatoes, which are rich in beta-carotene, a nutrient good for healthy skin and eyes. Adding to the gorgeous orange color, turmeric is touted for its anti-inflammatory properties.*

*Serves 4*

2 sweet potatoes, washed, skins on, sliced into ½ inch wide strips
2 T coconut oil or olive oil
1 t ground turmeric
1 t ground paprika
½ t salt
½ t freshly ground pepper

Preheat oven to 450°. Place the sweet potatoes on a baking sheet. Drizzle with the olive oil, turmeric, paprika, salt and pepper and toss with a spatula to combine. Roast for 30-40 minutes, turning potatoes once. They are done when brown and crisp at edges.

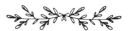

## ROASTED BEETROOT AND HORSERADISH ALMOND CREAM

*Beetroot or beets are an excellent source of vitamin C, fiber, and potassium. Whenever I make this dish, I also make the garlicky beet greens recipe that follows, or the Thai Noodles with Ginger Garlic Chicken (see the Excellent Entrees section) so I don't waste any of the beet plant or its nutrients. Beetroot greens, the tops to the beets, are a great source of phytonutrients.*

*Serves 6*

**3 large beets, washed, trimmed and unpeeled**
**Horseradish Almond Cream (see page 141)**
**2 T fresh oregano leaves or thyme**

Preheat oven to 400°. Fill a baking dish with one inch water. Place beets in water, and roast in oven for 45 minutes, until soft when poked with a knife. Allow beets to cool, then peel them under cold running water. Discard the skin. Cut the beets into small cubes. Place several spoonfuls of Horseradish Almond Cream onto individual plates. Top with beet cubes and sprinkle with oregano leaves to serve.

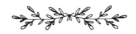

## GARLICKY BEET GREENS

*Beet greens are very high in antioxidants, vitamins, minerals, and fiber. It's a tragedy to throw them away! They are delicious sautéed in place of spinach or other greens.*

*Serves 2*

> 1 bunch beet greens, cut from beetroot, washed and dried well
> 2 T olive oil
> 1 clove garlic, chopped½ t salt
> Freshly ground pepper

Chop beet greens into 1" pieces. Place olive oil in a sauté pan. Add garlic and sauté over medium heat for 30 seconds. Add greens and salt and sauté until wilted. Add pepper to taste. Serve hot.

## ASIAN BROCCOLINI

*Broccolini is a hybrid of broccoli and Chinese broccoli. Sweeter and thinner than broccoli, broccolini is delicious on its own or tossed into Pasta. (See Pasta Primavera, page 187)*

*Serves 2-3*

> 1 large bunch broccolini
> 2 large cloves garlic, smashed
> 1 T olive oil

1 t ume plum vinegar, or more to taste*
1 t black sesame seeds

Wash broccolini and trim bottoms of stems. Slice thick stems lengthwise to make stems equal widths. Place olive oil in a sauté pan. Add garlic and sauté over medium heat for 30 seconds. Add broccolini and sauté for 2 to 3 minutes, or cooked through, but still bright green. Turn off heat. Add ume plum vinegar and sesame seeds and stir well. Serve hot.

*Technically a brine, not a vinegar, you can find ume plum vinegar in the Asian section of health food markets.

## ZUCCHINI "SOUFFLÉ"

*A simple and impressive side dish, this is the quickest way I know to turn a vegetable into soufflé.*

*Serves 6*

Drizzle olive oil
3 c zucchini, cubed (about 3 zucchini)
1 c Cashew Cream (see page 140)
4 eggs, slightly beaten
½ c onion, chopped
½ c olive oil
2 T parsley, chopped
3 cloves garlic, minced
½ t freshly ground pepper
¼ t salt

Preheat oven to 350°. Grease the bottom and sides of a 9 x 13" baking dish with the olive oil. In a medium bowl, combine all ingredients, then transfer to the baking dish, spreading evenly. Bake for 30 to 40 minutes or until edges are browned. Cut into squares. Serve warm.

## SPAGHETTI SQUASH

*Spaghetti squash is a great alternative to pasta. Providing iron, essential minerals, fiber and omega-3 fatty acids, spaghetti squash avoids the blood glucose spike that pasta causes. This recipe provides a simple way to roast and clean out the squash. Serve the cooked squash with your favorite pasta sauce or with garlic sautéed in olive oil and lemon.*

*Serves 3-4*

**1 medium size spaghetti squash**
**Olive oil**
**Pinch salt, optional**

Preheat oven to 375°. Carefully make 2 or 3 small slices into the top of the squash to allow steam to escape while baking. Place whole squash in a baking dish. Bake for 40-50 minutes until a knife easily slides through the outer skin. Allow to cool for a few minutes, then slice squash in half. Use fork to discard seeds and to loosen spaghetti-like strands. Place strands in a bowl, and, if desired, salt lightly before serving.

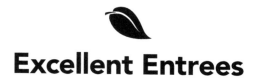

# Excellent Entrees

## GLUTEN-FREE CHICKEN NUGGETS

*Instead of flour or regular bread crumbs, these nuggets are rolled in gluten-free crumbs made from brown rice crisp cereal. When cooked, the cereal resembles crispy Panko in texture.*

*Serves 4*

> 2 lbs organic chicken breasts, skinned
> 2 eggs
> 2 c gluten-free "bread" crumbs (see page 142)
> 2 T olive oil

Preheat oven to 350°. Trim fat off chicken. Slice through each breast lengthwise to create two thin pieces, then cut each slice into squares about 1 ½ inches in size.

In a medium bowl, beat two eggs. In a large bowl, place the gluten-free "bread" crumbs. Add the chicken pieces to the eggs and stir, making sure each piece is well coated. Place coated chicken into the bowl with the crumbs and toss gently to make sure each piece is well coated.

Drizzle olive oil on a sheet pan, then use a spatula to evenly coat the bottom of the pan. Turn chicken out onto pan in a single layer. Cook for 20 minutes, flipping chicken once after the first 10 minutes. Test for doneness; chicken should be all white inside. Serve hot.

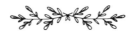

## BROCCOLI BAKED CHICKEN

*With the ghee, flour, and broth, this gluten- and dairy-free version of béchamel sauce makes this dish very moist and excellent served with rice.*

*Serves 4-6*

> 3 T ghee or olive oil, divided, plus extra to grease pans
> 3 organic chicken breasts
> 2 T onion, chopped
> 2 garlic cloves, minced
> 1 head broccoli florets
> 3 T gluten-free flour (see page 142)
> 2 ½ c low sodium chicken broth
> ¼ lb mushrooms, sliced
> 1 t fresh rosemary, chopped
> 1 t salt

Preheat oven to 375°. Grease a shallow 9" square baking dish with a bit of the extra ghee. Place 1 tablespoon of the ghee or olive oil into a large sauté pan. Add chicken breasts, onions, and garlic to pan. Sauté over medium heat for about 5 minutes, stirring vegetables occasionally. Turn chicken over, cover pan and continue cooking for another 5 minutes or until just cooked through. Remove chicken and slice on cutting board into ½ inch slices. Add to baking dish.

Meanwhile, in a steamer pot, or using steam insert in a saucepan, heat 1 inch of water to boiling. Add broccoli florets to steamer. Cover and steam for 5 minutes. Remove broccoli and place in baking dish.

Rinse the saucepan and reuse to melt the 2 remaining tablespoons of ghee or olive oil. Stir in the flour. Turn heat to low and add broth, stirring as it begins to thicken. Add mushrooms, rosemary, and salt to saucepan and cook for 5 minutes until mushrooms soften. Pour the mushroom sauce over the chicken and broccoli. Bake uncovered for 15 minutes. Serve hot.

## BOUILLABAISSE

*This recipe lends itself to variations. To turn it into an Italian Cioppino, use oregano as the herb and add more tomatoes. Or, to turn Bouillabaisse into Spanish Zarzuela, add ground almonds. Feel free to enjoy the shellfish with your hands. Serve with brown rice or brown rice pasta.*

*Serves 4-6*

1 clove garlic, minced
½ t freshly ground pepper
⅛ t saffron
2 T chopped fresh herbs such as basil, tarragon, or dill
3 T olive oil
1 onion, diced
1 tomato, chopped
2 lbs shellfish rinsed: one lobster tail per person cut open on underside, 3 shrimp in shells per person, 1 mussel per person or substitute clams, scallops or oysters
1 lb fresh fish steaks or fillets such as cod, halibut, and/or salmon, cut into bite-sized cubes
1 c dry white wine

In a small bowl, combine garlic, pepper, saffron, and herbs. Heat olive oil over low heat in a stockpot. Add herb/saffron mixture, onions and tomato. Cover pot and simmer for five minutes.

Add lobster first to bottom of the pot. Cover and cook for 3 minutes. Then add the shellfish to the bottom of pan and the fish on top of the shellfish. Add wine, cover pot, and bring liquid to a boil. Quickly reduce heat and simmer for 7 minutes, stirring occasionally, until fish is cooked through.

## TURKEY CHILI

*This chili makes a great and hearty meal served with brown rice and a salad or spooned over pasta.*

*Serves 4*

> 1 T olive oil
> 1 yellow onion, chopped
> 3 carrots, cleaned and chopped into bite size pieces
> 2 ribs celery, cleaned and chopped into bite size pieces
> 1 ½ lbs ground turkey
> 1 can black or pinto beans, drained and rinsed
> ½ t cumin, ground
> 1 t coriander, ground
> 1 t cinnamon, ground
> ½ t sea salt
> ½ t freshly ground black pepper
> 1 16 oz jar tomatillo salsa
> 1 15 oz container fresh tomato salsa
> ½ c Herbed Almond Cream (see page 140)
> 1 c cilantro, chopped

Heat olive oil in a sauté pan. Add onion, carrots and celery and cook over medium low heat for 5 minutes, or until onion becomes translucent. Add turkey and break apart with a spoon, stirring until cooked through, 8-10 minutes. Add beans, cumin, coriander, cinnamon, salt and pepper. Stir until well combined. Add both salsas. Stir well and cover. Continue cooking on medium low heat for 5-10 minutes. To serve, divide chili among bowls, then add a dollop of almond cream and lots of cilantro to each.

## THAI NOODLES WITH GINGER GARLIC CHICKEN

*This dish has lots of fresh ginger, which is a wonderful anti-inflammatory digestive aid. Tamari is a gluten-free soy sauce; organic is best to avoid GMO soy.*

*Serves 4*

For the chicken:
 Juice of 1 lime
 1 ½ T tamari or gluten-free soy sauce
 1 T fish sauce
 2 T maple syrup
 1 T olive oil
 1 t turmeric, ground
 2 cloves garlic, grated
 ½ t crushed red pepper flakes
 3 chicken breast halves, cut into 1" strips

For the noodles and veggies:
 1 16 oz package brown rice fettuccini or Pad Thai noodles
 1 T sesame oil

1 T olive oil
1 package fresh crimini mushrooms, sliced
1 large head bok choy, washed and chopped
Beet greens from 3 or more beets, washed well and
chopped
1 bunch scallions, thinly sliced
2 T fresh ginger, peeled and grated
1-2 T Sriracha sauce
1 c cilantro leaves, chopped
½ c mint leaves

In a large mixing bowl, combine all chicken ingredients and marinate chicken for ½ hour in fridge as you prepare the rest of the recipe.

Meanwhile, fill a pasta pot with water and bring to a boil. Cook noodles according to package directions. When noodles are done, strain and rinse with cold water.

While noodles cook, put sesame and olive oils into large sauté pan and warm over medium heat. Add mushrooms and sauté for 5 minutes, stirring and turning once or twice. Add bok choy, beet greens, scallions, and ginger and cook over medium-high heat for another 3 minutes. Add Sriracha, cilantro, and mint. Stir well to combine and heat through. Turn off heat and transfer veggies into a serving bowl along with cooked noodles. Stir well to coat noodles.

In same sauté pan, cook marinated chicken and sauce for 3-4 minutes; flip chicken and continue cooking until just cooked through, another 3 minutes. When done, add chicken and sauce to noodles, and stir well to combine. Serve hot.

## ASIAN QUINOA VEGGIE BOWL

*Since quinoa is very high in protein, this can be served as a veggie entrée or a side dish. Tamari is a gluten-free soy sauce; organic is best to avoid GMO soy.*

*Serves 3 as a main course*

- ½ c white quinoa
- ½ c red quinoa
- 1 t ground turmeric
- 1 t paprika
- 1 t ground cardamom
- 1 t dried onion flakes
- 1 t garlic powder
- ½ t salt
- 1 T olive oil
- 1 head broccoli, cut into long florets
- ⅓ lb green beans, cut into 1- to 2-inch pieces
- 2 c spinach leaves
- Salt and pepper
- 2 T Tamari sauce or gluten free soy sauce
- 2 T rice vinegar
- 1 T olive oil
- 1 T toasted sesame oil
- 1 t fresh ginger, peeled and grated
- 3 scallions, thinly sliced on the diagonal
- 2 t sesame seeds, toasted

Rinse both quinoas together in a colander. Place in a saucepan and cover with 2 cups of water. Add the turmeric, paprika, cardamom, onion flakes, garlic powder and salt. Cover and bring to a boil. Reduce heat to simmer and continue cooking for 12 minutes.

Heat olive oil in a sauté pan. Add broccoli and sauté over medium heat, for 5 minutes, stirring occasionally. Add green beans and continue cooking for 3 minutes, stirring to be sure veggies cook evenly. Add spinach leaves and cook for 2 more minutes, until just wilted. Add a pinch of salt and pepper to the veggies and stir. Turn off heat.

In a large bowl, combine Tamari, vinegar, oils, and ginger. Add veggies to the bowl and toss well. Add scallions and sesame seeds and toss to combine. Serve veggies over quinoa.

## STUFFED PEPPERS

*Abundantly overflowing with goodness and health, this dish is as impressive for a party as it is for the body.*

*Serves 4*

> 1 c brown rice
> 4 large yellow or orange peppers
> 1 T olive oil
> 1 small yellow onion, chopped
> 1 stalk celery, chopped
> 6 crimini mushrooms chopped
> 1 lb ground chicken
> 28 oz can Muir Glen organic fire roasted tomatoes, or similar
> 1 jalapeno pepper, seeded and chopped
> 1 T cinnamon
> 1 T chili powder
> 1 T dried oregano
> 1 T dried parsley
> 1 t celery salt

**½ t freshly ground pepper**
**1 avocado, chopped**
**Handful cilantro, chopped**

Cook rice according to package directions. Meanwhile, preheat oven to 350°. Slice the tops off of the yellow peppers leaving about ½" rim so that the pepper tops become lids. Clean out inside of peppers, discarding seeds and white membranes. Place peppers and lids open face down on baking sheet. Bake peppers for 5 minutes until warm and slightly soft.

Heat olive oil in a large sauté pan. Add onions and sauté over medium heat until they begin to soften. Add celery and mushrooms and sauté until mushrooms are a bit browned. Add ground chicken. Continue cooking until chicken is cooked through. Add ½ can of the tomatoes and refrigerate the rest for another meal. Stir thoroughly to combine. Add jalapeno, cinnamon, chili powder, oregano, parsley, celery salt, and pepper. Stir and heat until bubbling. To serve, fill yellow peppers alternating with rice and chicken mixture until very full. Top with chopped avocado and cilantro. Serve with pepper lids on top.

## PASTA PRIMAVERA

*While this recipe calls for the inclusion of watercress and Asian Broccolini, another recipe from this book, any vegetables can be substituted. For great flavor, include the ume plum vinegar and garlic from the broccolini recipe if substituting vegetables.*

*Serves 3*

1 ½ packages gluten free pasta
3 T olive oil, divided
9 fresh tomatoes, roughly chopped
½ bunch Italian parsley, chopped
½ yellow onion, chopped
½ t salt
1 bunch watercress, finely chopped
Asian Broccolini (see page 176)

In a pasta pot, bring water to a boil water, add pasta and cook according to package directions. When done, drain pasta and return to pot. Add 2 tablespoons olive oil and mix well.

Meanwhile, combine tomatoes and parsley in a large serving bowl and set aside. Heat remaining olive oil in a sauté pan. Add onion and salt and sauté over medium heat until beginning to caramelize, about 5 minutes. Turn off heat. Add watercress to the pan and stir to wilt. Add pasta and watercress and onion mixture to the bowl with the tomatoes and parsley. Add the Asian Broccolini and toss to combine. Serve hot.

## EASY ROAST SALMON

*I recommend buying wild Alaskan salmon both for cooking and when eating out. Unfortunately, all Atlantic salmon is now farmed, which means the fish is likely to be living in unnatural conditions and treated with antibiotics accordingly. The resulting health effects are not as beneficial as wild salmon and may, in fact, be detrimental.*

*Serves 4*

2 lbs wild Alaskan salmon fillets, skin removed
Olive oil
Salt
Freshly cracked pepper

Preheat oven to 450°. Coat both sides of salmon with olive oil. Sprinkle both sides with salt and pepper. Heat a 12-inch oven-proof skillet over medium high heat for a few minutes. Place salmon in the skillet and leave untouched for 2 minutes to sear. Flip salmon and repeat on other side for 2 minutes. Turn off heat.

Carefully place hot pan in the center of the oven and roast for 5-7 minutes depending on thickness of salmon and preference for doneness. Thinner ends of salmon can be cut and removed sooner. Serve immediately.

## SALMON SALAD

*This is a quick way to use leftover Easy Roast Salmon, or you can make it from canned wild salmon.*

*Serves 2*

1 lb cooked wild salmon filet
or canned wild salmon
2 T Horseradish Almond Cream (see page 141)
2 stalks celery, chopped
1 t celery salt
1 t Herbs de Provence
1 T freshly squeezed lemon juice

In a medium bowl, mash salmon with fork, removing any small bones. Add remaining ingredients and combine well. Serve immediately or refrigerate for later.

## SOLE MEUNIÈRE

*This sole is a gluten-free, dairy-free twist on a classic French dish.*

*Serves 2*

> 1 T ghee
> 4 fillets of Dover or Petrale sole
> Gluten-free flour (see page 142)
> Juice of 1 lemon
> Salt
> 1 t capers
> 1 T parsley, finely chopped

Melt ghee in a large sauté pan and swirl to cover bottom of the pan. Add filets to pan side by side. Allow to cook for 3 minutes untouched. Flip filets gently with a spatula and cook for 2-3 minutes on the other side. While still cooking, drizzle lemon juice over fish, allowing juice to sizzle on bottom of pan. Sprinkle fish with salt, capers and parsley, and serve.

## CHICKEN SALAD

*Chicken salad is great to make the day after you've made the chicken soup on page 164. After the chicken has cooled in the refrigerator overnight, it is easy to shred. This dish can be served as a main course for dinner with a salad of arugula or romaine lettuce, or it can be part of a sandwich or lettuce wrap for lunch.*

*Serves 4*

> 3 chicken breasts cooked in chicken soup, removed from bone and shredded
> 1 T white wine vinegar
> 1 T rice wine vinegar
> 1 T lemon juice
> 2 T organic mayonnaise
> 1 T Dijon mustard
> ¼ c olive oil
> 1 celery stalk, chopped
> 1 c green or red grapes, sliced in half
> 2 T herb of choice, chopped (eg, fresh tarragon, thyme, mint)

In a medium bowl, combine all ingredients. Mix well, and serve.

## CHICKEN TOSTADAS

*Tostadas are another great way to use chicken cooked in the chicken soup recipe on page 164. In a pinch, you can also use a store-bought organic rotisserie chicken to make this dish.*

*Serves 4-6*

> 6 brown rice tortillas or all-veggie wraps
> 1 T olive oil
> ½ onion, chopped

1 red pepper, trimmed and sliced lengthwise
3 chicken breasts cooked in chicken soup, removed from
bone and shredded
2 scallions, trimmed and thinly sliced
1 tomato, chopped
1 avocado, chopped
½ c cilantro, chopped
Sriracha sauce or Pico de Gallo, to taste
1 lime, sliced into 6 wedges
Herbed Almond Cream (see page 140), optional

Heat oven to 350°. Place tortillas on cookie sheets in a single layer. Heat for 2 minutes until just warmed.

Warm olive oil in a sauté pan. Add onion and cook for 5 minutes over medium heat until translucent, stirring occasionally. Add pepper slices and shredded chicken and stir. Continue cooking until chicken edges begin to turn golden, about 5 minutes. Add scallions and cook for 2 minutes more. Remove pan from heat. Place each tortilla on a plate and spoon the chicken mixture on top. Sprinkle each tostada with tomato, avocado and cilantro. Serve with hot sauce, lime wedges and bowl of almond cream on the side.

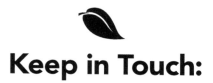

# Keep in Touch:

Don't miss a single thing! Sign up for my monthly news-letter for more mouth-watering recipes and health tips here: http://www.nanfosterhealth.com/newsletter-sign-up-page.html

**CONNECT WITH ME:**

On Facebook: https://www.facebook.com/nan.g.foster
By Email: nanfosterhealth@gmail.com
Website: www.nanfosterhealth.com

**HIRE ME FOR:**

Nutrition talks, cooking demos, one-on-one coaching

**REVIEW:**

Did you enjoy this book? I would love your review! Please give me your honest feedback on Amazon!

# Health Coach Training Program:

This book was inspired by my experience at the Institute for Integrative Nutrition® (IIN®) where I received my training in holistic wellness and health coaching.

IIN® offers a comprehensive Health Coach Training Program. From the physical aspects of nutrition and eating wholesome foods that work best for each individual person, to the concept of Primary Food–the idea that everything in life, including our spirituality, career, relationships, and fitness, contribute to our inner and outer health–IIN® helped me reach optimal health and balance. This inner journey unleashed the passion that compelled me to share what I've learned and to inspire others.

From renowned wellness experts as Visiting Teachers to the convenience of their online learning platform, this school has changed my life and I believe it will do the same for you. I invite you to learn more about the Institute for Integrative Nutrition® and explore how the Health Coach Training Program can help you transform your life.

Feel free to contact me to hear more about my personal experience at www.nanfosterhealth.com/integrativenutrition, or call (844) 315-8546 to learn more.

# REFERENCES

1. Jeffries, Matlock A., Mikhail Dozmorov, Yuhong Tang, Joan T. Merrill, Jonathan D. Wren, and Amr H. Sawalha. "Genome-wide DNA Methylation Patterns in CD4 T Cells from Patients with Systemic Lupus Erythematosus." 6.5 (2011): 593-601. *Epigenetics*. Landes Bioscience, May 2011. Web. 29 Feb. 2016. <http://www.ncbi.nlm.nih.gov/pmc/articles/PMC3121972/>.

2. Samsel, Anthony, and Stephanie Seneff. "Glyphosate, Pathways to Modern Diseases II: Celiac Sprue and Gluten Intolerance." *Interdisciplinary Toxicology* 6.4 (2013): 159-84. *Interdisciplinary Toxicology*. Slovak Toxicology Society SETOX, Dec. 2013. Web. 29 Feb. 2016.<http://www.ncbi.nlm.nih.gov/pmc/articles/PMC3945755/>.

3. Samsel, Anthony, and Stephanie Seneff. "Glyphosate's Suppression of Cytochrome P450 Enzymes and Amino Acid Biosynthesis by the Gut Microbiome: Pathways to Modern Diseases." *Entropy* 15.4 (2013): 1416-463. *MDPI*. Web. 29 Feb. 2016.<http://www.mdpi.com/1099-4300/15/4/1416>.

4. Galland, Leo, M.D. "Foundation for Integrated Medicine - LEAKY GUT SYNDROMES: BREAKING THE VICIOUS CYCLE" N.p., n.d. Web. 29 Feb. 2016. <http://www.mdheal.org/leakygut.htm>.

5. Hyman, Mark, M.D. "Think Yourself Thin? How About Think Yourself Well! - Dr. Mark Hyman." *Drhyman.com*. N.p., 5 Oct. 2015. Web. 29 Feb. 2016. <http://drhyman.com/blog/2014/10/30/think-thin-think-well/>.

6. Smith, Peter Andrey. "Can the Bacteria in Your Gut Explain Your Mood?" *The New York Times*. The New York Times, 27 June 2015. Web. 29 Feb. 2016. <http://www.nytimes.com/2015/06/28/magazine/can-the-bacteria-in-your-gut-explain-your-mood.html?_r=0>.

7. Mozaffarian, D., and EJ Benjamin, et al. "Heart Disease and Stroke Statistics–2015 Update: A Report from the American Heart Association." *Heart.org*. N.p., 17 Dec. 2014. Web. <https://www.heart.org/idc/groups/ahamah-public/@wcm/@sop/@smd/documents/downloadable/ucm_470704.pdf>.

8. *Report: Generation in Jeopardy.* Rep. N.p.: n.p., n.d.Pesticide Action Network North America, 2012. Web. 29 Feb. 2016. <http://www.panna.org/resources/publication-report/report-generation-jeopardy>.

9. Crimmins, Eileen M., and Hiram Beltrán-Sánchez. "Mortality and Morbidity Trends: Is There Compression of Morbidity?" *The Journals of Gerontology: Series B* 66.1 (2010): 75-86. Oxford University Press. Web. 29 Feb. 2016. <http://psychsocgerontology.oxfordjournals.org/content/66B/1/75.short>.

10. Ava, Miriam. "Gratitude Speaks: Dr. Mario Martinez, Author of the No. 1 Bestselling 'The MindBody Code'" *The Huffington Post.* TheHuffingtonPost.com, 27 May 2015. Web. 29 Feb. 2016. <http://www.huffingtonpost.com/miriam-ava/gratitude-speaks-dr-mario_b_7302106.html>.

11. Pert, Candace B., Ph.D. *Molecules of Emotion: The Science Behind Mind-Body Medicine.* New York: Scribner, 1997. Print.

12. Myers, Wendy. "Food Sensitivities Make You Fat and Sick - Liveto110.com." *Live to 110.* N.p., n.d. Web. 29 Feb. 2016. <https://liveto110.com/food-sensitivities-make-you-fat-and-sick/>.

13. Mercola, Joseph, D.O. "Welcome to the Beginner Nutrition Plan." *Mercola.com.* N.p., n.d. Web. 29 Feb. 2016. <http://www.mercola.com/nutritionplan/beginner.htm>.

14. Jackson, KD, LD Howie, and LJ Akinbami. *Trends in Allergic Conditions among Children: United States, 1997-2011.* NCHS Data Brief, No 121. Hyattsville, MD: National Center for Health Statistics, 2013. Web. <http://www.cdc.gov/nchs/data/databriefs/db121.pdf>

15. Orbach, Hiram, N. Agmon-Levin, and G. Zandman-Goddard. "Vaccines and Autoimmune Diseases of the Adult." *Discovery Medicine* 9.45 (2010): 90-97. *National Center for Biotechnology Information.* U.S. National Library of Medicine. Web. 29 Feb. 2016. <http://www.ncbi.nlm.nih.gov/pubmed/20193633>.

16. Ercolini, A. M., and S. D. Miller. "The Role of Infections in Autoimmune Disease." *Clinical and Experimental Immunology* 15.1 (2009): 1-15. NCBI. Web. 29 Feb. 2016. <http://www.ncbi.nlm.nih.gov/pmc/articles/PMC2665673/>.

17. Hyman, Mark, MD. "Helpful or the Latest Fad? The Truth About Detoxification - Dr. Mark Hyman." *Dr Mark Hyman.* N.p., 07 Mar. 2015. Web. 29 Feb. 2016. <http://drhyman.com/blog/2015/03/07/truth-about-detoxification/>.

18. Smith, Jeffrey M. "Are Genetically Modified Foods a Gut-Wrenching Combination?" *ResponsibleTechnology.org.* N.p., n.d. Web. <http://responsibletechnology.org/glutenintroduction/>.

19. Ornish, D, MJ Magbanua, and G. Weidner. "Changes in Prostate Gene Expression in Men Undergoing an Intensive Nutrition and Lifestyle Intervention." *Proc Natl Acad Sci* 105.24 (2008): 8369-374. *National Center for Biotechnology Information.* U.S. National Library of Medicine, 16 June 2008. Web. 29 Feb. 2016. <http://www.ncbi.nlm.nih.gov/pubmed/18559852>.

20. Chopra, Deepak, MD. "How Your Genes Can Make You Happier." *Chopra.com.* The Chopra Center, n.d. Web. 29 Feb. 2016. <http://www.chopra.com/ccl/how-your-genes-can-make-you-happier>.

21. Akcay, MN, and G. Akcay. "The Presence of the Antigliadin Antibodies in Autoimmune Thyroid Diseases." *Hepatogastroenterology* 50.2 (2003): Cclxxix-clxxx. *National Center for Biotechnology Information.* U.S. National Library of Medicine. Web. 29 Feb. 2016. <http://www.ncbi.nlm.nih.gov/pubmed/15244201>.

22. Ayers, Art, Ph.D. "Contagious Health." *Cooling Inflammation.* N.p., 1 June 2011. Web. 29 Feb. 2016. <http://coolinginflammation.blogspot.com/2011/06/contagious-health.html>.

23. Segersten, Alissa. "How to Optimize Your Digestion for a Large Meal." *Whole Life Nutrition®.* N.p., n.d. Web. 29 Feb. 2016. <https://wholelifenutrition.net/articles/digestive-health/how-optimize-your-digestion-large-meal#sthash.zp3Bx2uo.dpuf>.

24. Woodyard, Catherine. "Exploring the Therapeutic Effects of Yoga and Its Ability to Increase Quality of Life." *International Journal of Yoga* 4.2 (2011): 49-54. *International Journal of Yoga.* Medknow Publications Pvt Ltd. Web. 31 Mar. 2016. <http://www.ncbi.nlm.nih.gov/pmc/articles/PMC3193654/>.

25. Lally, Phillippa, C. Van Jaarsveld, H. Potts, and J. Wardle. "How Are Habits Formed: Modelling Habit Formation in the Real World." *European Journal of Social Psychology Eur. J. Soc. Psychol.* 40.6 (2009): 998-1009. Web. 29 Feb. 2016. <http://onlinelibrary.wiley.com/doi/10.1002/ejsp.674/abstract>.

# RESOURCES

# FOOD FAVORITES

## CHOOSE CLEAN, NUTRIENT-DENSE FOODS

- ANDI scale, Joel Fuhrman, MD, https://www.drfuhrman.com/library/andi-food-scores.aspx
- NuVal, David Katz, MD, https://www.nuval.com
- Clean 15 and Dirty Dozen, Environmental Working Group, www.ewg.org

# MOOD FAVORITES

## ALTERNATIVE THERAPIES

- **Acupuncture** is used to treat many stress-related conditions including autoimmune diseases, blood pressure, hormone balance, anxiety, and depression. Find a practitioner in your area.
- **Eye Movement Desensitization Reprogramming (EMDR)**, originally used to treat PTSD, is a form of

integrative psychotherapy for the relief of trauma, incorporating many therapy modalities. Find a practitioner in your area.

- **Emotional Freedom Technique**, also called Tapping, is used to reprogram our thoughts and emotions combining energy meridians from acupuncture, as well as neuro-linguistic programming and Thought Field Therapy. Visit http://www.thetappingsolution.com
- **Guided meditation**. There are many guided meditations online. Some examples to explore (search for them on the internet) are those from:
  - Jack Kornfield
  - Chopra Center
  - Eckhart Tolle
  - Holosync by Centerpointe, an audio technology inducing brain wave patterns of deep meditation

# GLOSSARY

**ADD, ADHD** (Attention Deficit Disorder and Attention Deficit Hyperactivity Disorder): Typically seen in children, but affecting adults as well, ADD is a condition of inattentiveness, dreaminess, impulsiveness, and short attention span. It can be associated with learning disorders and with hyperactivity (ADHD), and is not caused by any known underlying mental or physical disorder.

**Arthritis**: Inflammation and stiffness in joints that typically worsens with age. There are two types of arthritis: osteoarthritis, which causes cartilage to break down and rheumatoid arthritis, an autoimmune disease, which attacks the joint lining. Other autoimmune diseases such as lupus can cause additional types of joint inflammation.

**Celiac disease**: An autoimmune disease that triggers a response to gluten in the small intestine. The villi, or small finger like projections on the lining of the intestine, become flattened and incapable of properly absorbing nutrients. Diagnosis is made by endoscopy.

**Crohn's disease**: An autoimmune disease causing inflammation of the small and large intestine. Crohn's can be mild or severe and can lead to erosions to the inner lining, scarring, stiffness, narrowing, and obstruction of the bowel. Common symptoms include diarrhea, vomiting, and weight loss. Diagnosis is made by x-ray or colonoscopy.

**Eczema**: An autoimmune inflammatory condition affecting the skin characterized by red, scaly patches and blisters that can become rough, blistered, itchy, and oozing. Eczema is seen in about 10 to 20 percent of infants in the U.S. and approximately three percent of adults and children.

**Fibromyalgia**: An autoimmune disease characterized by chronic pain and intermittent tenderness in muscles, joints, and tendons. The condition can be accompanied by fatigue, memory, mood, sleep, and anxiety issues.

**Graves' disease**: An autoimmune disease causing hyperthyroid activity. With Graves' disease, thyroid-stimulating antibodies cause the thyroid gland to grow and produce too much thyroid hormone. Graves' is seen more frequently in women.

**Gut dysbiosis**: An imbalance of gut flora in the digestive tract with an overgrowth of bad bacteria and too few beneficial bacteria. Under normal circumstances, the flora contains 85 percent beneficial bacteria and 15 percent bad bacteria. The beneficial bacteria aid in digestion and immune regulation. Under certain conditions, this microbial ratio can become imbalanced causing gas, bloating, diarrhea, constipation, fatigue, brain fog, and a diagnosis of Irritable Bowel Syndrome (IBS).

**Hashimoto's thyroiditis**: An inflammation of the thyroid gland caused by attacks from wayward immune system cells producing decreased thyroid hormone and, possibly, goiter. The most common form of hypothyroidism, Hashimoto's affects women seven times more often than men and causes such symptoms as fatigue, hair loss, weight gain, dry skin, and sensitivity to cold.

**Immune system**: The body's defense system that recognizes that which is "self" versus that which is foreign under normal circumstances and attacks foreign invaders. The immune system is comprised of a multitude of tissues and cells including the thymus gland, spleen, and lymph nodes, specialized tissue in the digestive tract and bone marrow, and cells including macrophages and lymphocytes (antibodies, B cells, and T cells).

**Irritable Bowel Syndrome** (IBS): A very common condition estimated to affect between 25 and 45 million Americans. While it is a non-inflammatory condition, it can cause the same symptoms as the Inflammatory Bowel Disease, including diarrhea, constipation, abdominal pain, and cramps.

**Irritable Bowel Disease** (IBD). A term for a range of conditions that cause inflammation of the intestines. These conditions include Crohn's disease, ulcerative colitis, and other forms of colitis, and affect as many as 1.4 million Americans. Unlike IBS, IBD is characterized as a disease. In addition to the abdominal symptoms of IBS, IBD can cause a range of symptoms including eye discomfort, extreme fatigue, joint pain, and rectal bleeding,

**Leaky gut:** A permeability of the lining of the digestive tract characterized by a loosening of the tight junctions in the gut that normally keep food particles contained within the gut. There are many possible causes of leaky gut including toxins, alcohol, gut dysbiosis, parasites, gluten, and non-steroidal anti-inflammatory drugs (NSAIDs) among others.

**Lupus (System Lupus Erythematosus):** An autoimmune disease causing chronic inflammation. The inflammation can affect many different areas of the body including joints, muscles, skin, kidneys, blood cells, brain, heart, and lungs. A key characteristic of lupus is a butterfly-shaped rash across both cheeks.

**Microbiome:** A symbiotic community of microorganisms, such as bacteria and fungi, living in a particular environment, particularly on and in nasal passages, oral cavities, skin, urogenital tract and gastrointestinal tract of the human body. The gut microbiome contains 100 trillion diverse colonies of microbes that protect us from harmful germs and help break down food for digestion and nutrient absorption.

**Multiple sclerosis:** An chronic autoimmune disease affecting the nerves of the central nervous system including the brain, spinal cord, and optic nerves, and causing numerous symptoms throughout the body. The immune system attacks the myelin sheath, the insulation around nerves that aids in communication between the brain and the body. The nerve fibers themselves are vulnerable to scarring and permanent damage.

**Pemphigus vulgaris**: A less common autoimmune disease. Antibiodies attack specific proteins in the skin and mucus membranes causing blisters in the mouth, scalp, and other areas on the skin. Pemphigus typically affects those who are middle aged and older.

**Perniosis**: Also known as chilblains, perniosis is an inflammatory condition affecting the small blood vessels in skin. During exposure to cold air and dampness, the condition can cause itching, redness, painful swelling, and blistering primarily on the hands, feet, and face. Unlike frostbite, perniosis is a sensitivity to cold which can be often be resolved with proper exercise and diet.

**Psoriasis**: A common chronic inflammatory skin condition that causes the build-up of extra skin cells. Characterized by scaly red patches covered with silvery scales that can by itchy, dry, and painful, psoriasis is not contagious.

**Raynaud's Syndrome**: More common in women than men, Raynaud's is a condition of blood vessel constriction primarily in fingers and toes when one is exposed to cold or under emotional stress. This vasoconstriction causes discomfort in the extremities and a blue or white discoloration. Raynaud's occurs most commonly on its own as a primary condition, or as a secondary condition in association with other disorders such as connective tissue disorders and autoimmune diseases.

**Rheumatoid arthritis**: The most common form of autoimmune arthritis, it affects about 1.3 million people in the U.S., most commonly in women over age 40. The immune system attacks the lining of joints primarily in hands and feet causing painful inflammation. Over time, this inflammation can lead to joint bone erosion and joint disfigurement. By comparison, osteo-arthritis, which affects millions, is the most common form of arthritis and occurs from a wearing down of cartilage in joints.

**Rosacea**: A chronic skin condition causing redness, frequently with red bumps, on the face. It is often mistaken for acne and affects approximately 14 million people in the U.S.

**Serum sickness**: An immune response to certain medications or to the administration of antiserum–the liquid part of blood containing antibodies provided as protection against germs and toxins. Similar to an allergy, serum sickness reactions include fever, rash, enlarged lymph nodes, arthritis, and joint pain.

**Sjogren's disease:** A chronic inflammatory autoimmune condition in which the immune system attacks mucous membranes and glands of the eyes and mouth that secrete moisture resulting in decreased tears and saliva. More common in women over age 40, Sjogren's can strike at any age and frequently occurs along with other autoimmune conditions such as lupus.

**Type 1 diabetes**: Typically diagnosed in people under age 20, Type 1 diabetes is an autoimmune condition affecting about 5 percent of people with diabetes. The immune system attacks the cells that produce insulin in the pancreas, called the beta cells. This results in little to no insulin production and an inability to use glucose for energy. Chronic high glucose levels can cause atherosclerosis and damage nerves and blood vessels in the kidneys, eyes, and heart.

**Type 2 diabetes**: Unlike Type 1 diabetes, Type 2 is not an auto-immune disease. Rather, it is caused by chronic high blood sugar levels and a resulting insensitivity to insulin. As a result, blood glucose cannot be used for energy, and blood sugar levels increase leading to hyperglycemia. While Type 2 diabetes occurs most frequently hand-in-hand with obesity, it is also more common in certain ethnicities including blacks, American Indians, and Asian Americans. More common in those over 45, incidence of Type 2 diabetes is climbing among children and teens due to childhood obesity.

## ABOUT THE AUTHOR

Nan Foster's background in biology and psychology, her love of cooking, and her sudden diagnosis of lupus in her late 30's provided the foundations for her discovery of a disease-reversing food-mood method and her subsequent career as a health coach. She takes clients on a journey of self-discovery, and lovingly fosters gradual changes to help them improve wellness, vitality, and joy. Nan works with people who are stressed, fatigued, inflamed, and motivated to embrace healthful habits. Clients describe her as "compassionate," "insightful," and "inspiring."

Nan helped launch the nation's first 100 percent organic, non-GMO school lunch program. She has written for *Self*, *Glamour*, and *Avenue* magazines, and on behalf of numerous companies in the biotechnology and life sciences industries. Her interest in mind-body health dates back to her days at Vassar College. For more information on Nan, visit www.NanFosterHealth.com.

10960261R00116

Made in the USA
Lexington, KY
08 October 2018